The Complete Plant-Based

Cookbook for Beginners

2000+ Days of easy and Delicious Vegan Recipes for Nourishing Your Body and Mind. Incl. 30 Days Meal Plan to Help You Embrace the Love for Vegan Diet

Samuel Sousa

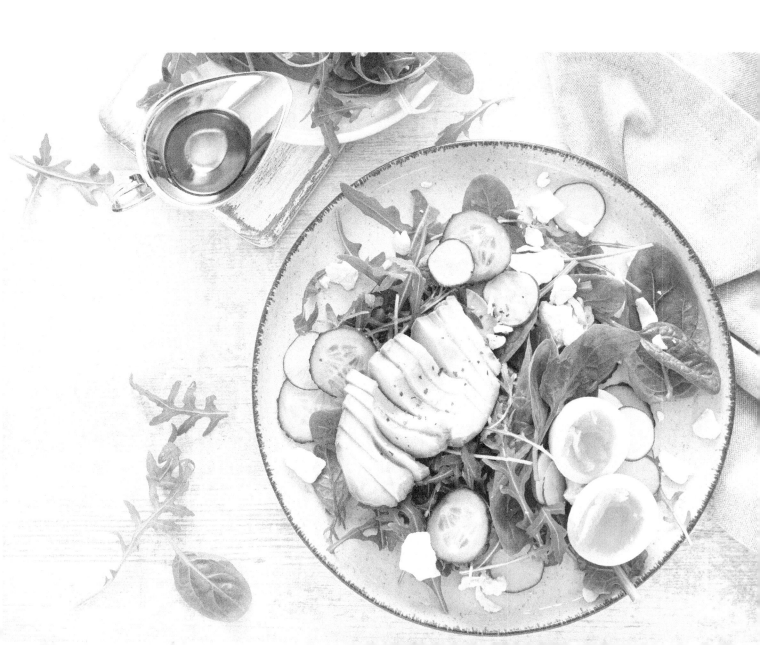

Table of Contents

Chapter 5 Beans and Grains

Chapter 6 Snacks and Appetizers

Chapter 7 Vegetables and Sides 54

Chapter 8 Desserts 63

Chapter 9 Stews and Soups 71

Chapter 11 Staples, Sauces, Dips, and Dressings   91

Appendix 1: Measurement Conversion Chart   101

Appendix 2: The Dirty Dozen and Clean Fifteen   102

INTRODUCTION

Welcome to a culinary journey that celebrates the power and beauty of plant-based eating. In this cookbook, we invite you to explore the remarkable world of plant-based cuisine and discover the endless possibilities it offers for nourishing your body, expanding your palate, and embracing a sustainable lifestyle.

In recent years, there has been a remarkable shift in the way people approach their dietary choices. More individuals are recognizing the tremendous benefits of adopting a plant-based diet, not only for their own health but also for the well-being of the planet. By choosing to center our meals around plant-based ingredients, we unlock a world of flavors, textures, and culinary creativity that can transform the way we eat and live.

The health benefits of a plant-based diet are well-documented. Studies have shown that a plant-based eating pattern can reduce the risk of chronic diseases, including heart disease, diabetes, and certain types of cancer. By prioritizing whole, unprocessed foods derived from plants, such as fruits, vegetables, legumes, whole grains, nuts, and seeds, we provide our bodies with a rich array of essential nutrients, antioxidants, and fiber that support optimal health and vitality.

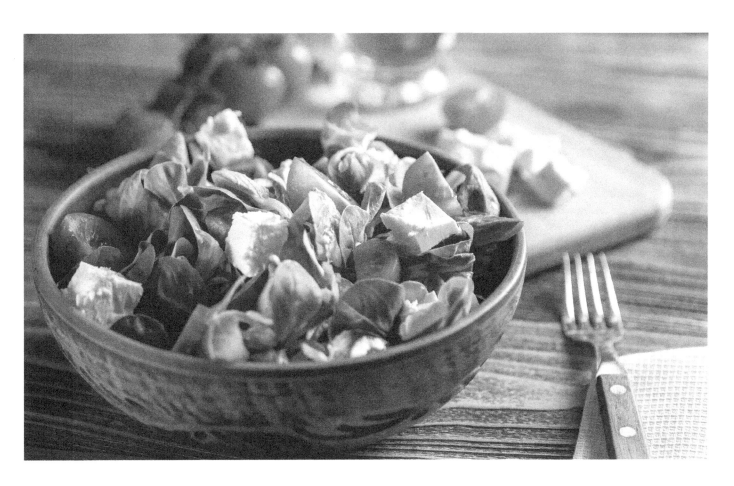

Beyond personal well-being, embracing a plant-based diet has profound implications for the health of our planet. Animal agriculture, with its significant land, water, and resource requirements, contributes to deforestation, greenhouse gas emissions, and biodiversity loss. By shifting towards plant-based eating, we reduce our ecological footprint and contribute to the preservation of our environment for future generations. It's a powerful way to make a positive impact on the world around us.

In this cookbook, we aim to inspire and empower you to embrace the incredible flavors and possibilities of plant-based eating. From vibrant salads and hearty soups to satisfying main dishes and delectable desserts, our carefully crafted recipes showcase the versatility and creativity of plant-based cuisine. Whether you're an experienced cook or just starting your culinary journey, you'll find a wealth of delicious options that will tempt your taste buds and nourish your body.

We also provide practical guidance on key aspects of a plant-based lifestyle, including essential pantry ingredients, helpful cooking techniques, and tips for meal planning and preparation. We address common questions and concerns, ensuring that you feel confident and supported as you navigate this exciting culinary adventure.

So, join us on this journey to vibrant health and delicious flavors. Let's celebrate the abundance of nature's bounty and discover the incredible potential of plant-based eating. Together, we can create a more sustainable and compassionate world, one delicious meal at a time. Get ready to be inspired, empowered, and transformed by the power of plants.

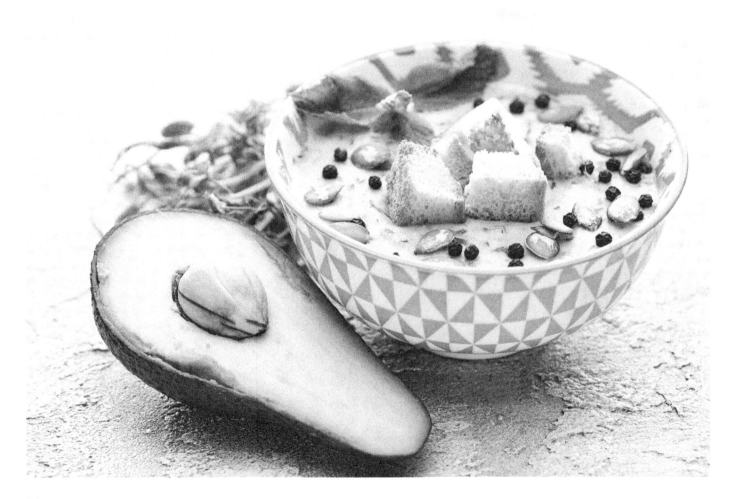

Chapter 1 The Power of Plant-Based Eating

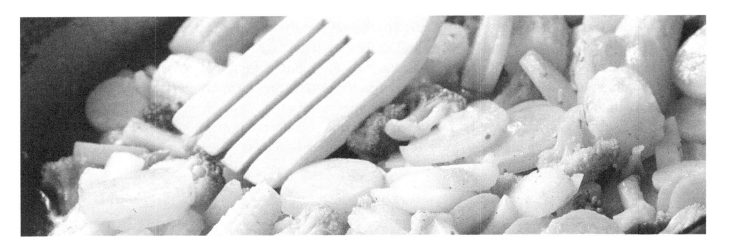

Health Benefits of a Plant-Based Diet

A plant-based diet offers a wide range of health benefits due to its emphasis on whole, unprocessed plant foods. Here are some key health benefits associated with a plant-based diet:

Reduced Risk of Chronic Diseases: Numerous studies have shown that a plant-based diet is associated with a lower risk of chronic diseases such as heart disease, high blood pressure, type 2 diabetes, and certain types of cancer. The high fiber content, abundant antioxidants, and phytochemicals found in plant foods contribute to these protective effects.

Heart Health: Plant-based diets are typically low in saturated fat and cholesterol while being rich in heart-healthy nutrients like fiber, antioxidants, and unsaturated fats. This combination helps to lower blood cholesterol levels, reduce inflammation, improve blood pressure, and support overall cardiovascular health.

Weight Management: Plant-based diets are generally lower in calories and higher in fiber compared to diets rich in animal products. The high fiber content helps to promote feelings of fullness and satisfaction, which can aid in weight management

and reduce the risk of obesity.

Improved Digestive Health: Plant-based diets are naturally high in fiber, which promotes regular bowel movements, prevents constipation, and supports a healthy digestive system. Additionally, the abundance of antioxidants and anti-inflammatory compounds found in plant foods can help reduce the risk of digestive disorders, such as diverticulitis and inflammatory bowel disease.

Enhanced Nutrient Intake: A well-planned plant-based diet can provide an array of essential nutrients, including vitamins, minerals, and phytochemicals. By consuming a diverse range of plant foods, individuals can meet their nutrient needs and benefit from the synergistic effects of these various compounds.

Better Blood Sugar Control: Plant-based diets, particularly those rich in whole grains, legumes, fruits, and vegetables, have been shown to improve insulin sensitivity and blood sugar control. This can be particularly beneficial for individuals with type 2 diabetes or those at risk of developing the condition.

Lower Risk of Obesity: Plant-based diets tend to be lower in calorie density, meaning they provide fewer calories per gram of food. This can help individuals achieve and maintain a healthy weight, reducing the risk of obesity and associated health problems.

Anti-Inflammatory Effects: Many plant foods possess anti-inflammatory properties due to their high content of antioxidants and phytochemicals. By reducing chronic inflammation in the body, a plant-based diet can help prevent and manage conditions such as arthritis, autoimmune diseases, and certain cancers.

Improved Gut Microbiome: Plant-based diets, rich in fiber and prebiotics, can promote a diverse and healthy gut microbiome. A balanced and diverse gut microbiome is associated with improved digestion, nutrient absorption, immune function, and mental health.

Longevity and Overall Well-Being: Studies have suggested that individuals who follow a plant-based diet may have a longer lifespan and better overall well-being. This may be attributed to the positive effects on health markers, reduced risk of chronic diseases, and the consumption of nutrient-dense, whole foods.

It's important to note that while a plant-based diet can provide significant health benefits, it's essential to plan meals carefully to ensure adequate intake of essential nutrients, such as vitamin B12, iron, calcium, and omega-3 fatty acids. Consulting with a registered dietitian or healthcare professional can help ensure you're meeting your specific nutritional needs while following a plant-based diet.

Environmental Impact of Food Choices

The environmental impact of our food choices is a critical consideration in today's world. The food we consume has a significant effect on the environment, including climate change, land use, water resources, and biodiversity. Here are some key points highlighting the environmental impact of food choices:

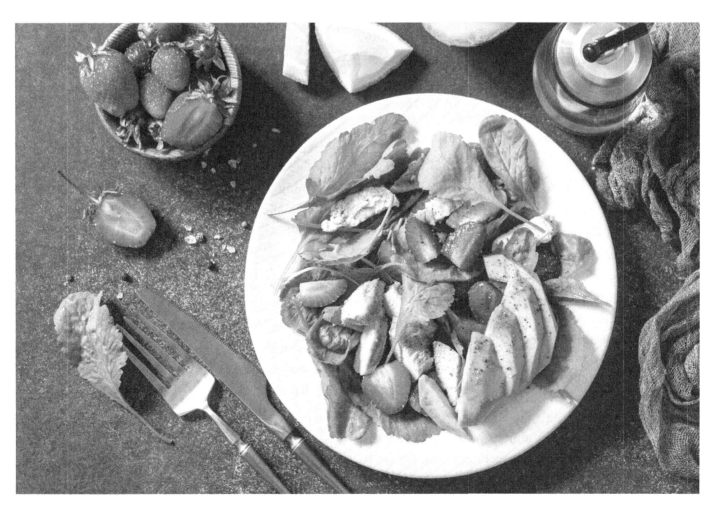

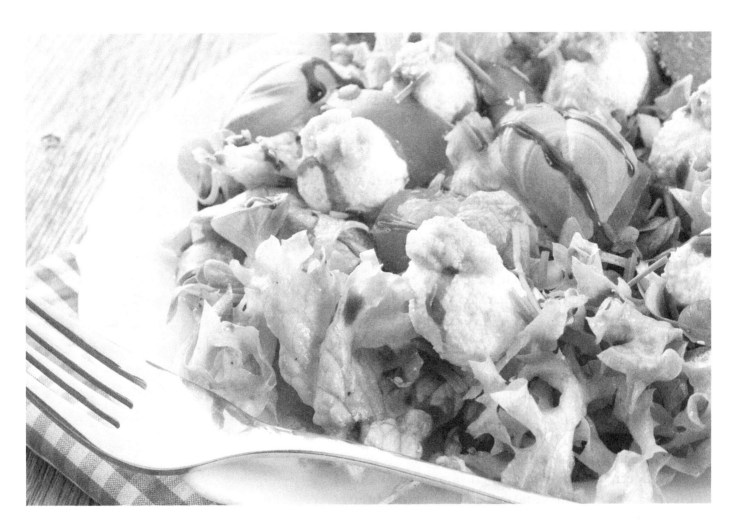

Greenhouse Gas Emissions: The production of animal-based foods, particularly meat and dairy products, is a major contributor to greenhouse gas emissions. Livestock farming, especially industrial-scale operations, releases significant amounts of methane, a potent greenhouse gas. By choosing plant-based foods, we can reduce our carbon footprint and contribute to mitigating climate change.

Land Use and Deforestation: Animal agriculture requires vast amounts of land for grazing and growing animal feed crops. The expansion of livestock farming often leads to deforestation, which contributes to habitat loss, biodiversity decline, and increased greenhouse gas emissions. Choosing plant-based foods reduces the demand for land-intensive animal farming and helps protect forests and natural ecosystems.

Water Consumption: Animal agriculture is a water-intensive industry. It requires substantial amounts of water for animal drinking, irrigation of feed crops, and cleaning facilities. In contrast, plant-based foods generally have a lower water footprint. By opting for plant-based options, we can conserve water resources and reduce the strain on freshwater ecosystems.

Pollution and Water Quality: Livestock farming can contribute to water pollution through the release of excess nutrients, pesticides, and antibiotics into waterways. The runoff from animal farms can contaminate rivers, lakes, and coastal areas, causing harmful algal blooms and disrupting aquatic ecosystems. Choosing plant-based foods reduces the environmental pollution associated with intensive animal agriculture.

Energy Consumption: The production, processing, and transportation of animal-based foods require significant energy inputs. This includes energy used for animal feed production, livestock farming operations, and refrigeration. Plant-based diets tend to have a lower energy demand, contributing to overall energy conservation and reduced reliance on fossil fuels.

Food Waste: Food waste is a significant environmental issue. Choosing plant-based foods can help reduce food waste since plant-based ingredients often have a longer shelf life compared to perishable animal products. By minimizing food waste, we can reduce the environmental impact associated with food production, including wasted resources such as water, land, and energy.

Sustainable Agriculture: Plant-based diets align well with sustainable agriculture practices. Organic farming, regenerative agriculture, and agroecological approaches often prioritize plant-based food production, emphasizing soil health, biodiversity conservation, and reduced chemical inputs. By supporting sustainable agricultural practices, we can promote environmental stewardship and protect natural resources.

Conservation of Biodiversity: Animal agriculture can contribute to habitat destruction and the loss of biodiversity. Choosing plant-based foods reduces the demand for animal farming, which, in turn, can help preserve habitats and protect endangered species. By promoting biodiversity conservation, we support the resilience of ecosystems and ensure the long-term sustainability of our planet.

Considering the environmental impact of our food choices is crucial for creating a sustainable future. Transitioning to a plant-based diet, even partially, can significantly reduce our ecological footprint and contribute to a healthier planet. By making informed and conscious decisions about the foods we consume, we can support a more sustainable and environmentally friendly food system.

Ethical Considerations of a Plant-Based Lifestyle

Adopting a plant-based lifestyle goes beyond personal health and environmental concerns. It also raises important ethical considerations related to animal welfare, compassion, and our moral responsibility towards other living beings. Here are some key ethical considerations associated with a plant-based lifestyle:

Animal Welfare: Many individuals choose a plant-based lifestyle out of concern for the well-being and ethical treatment of animals. Factory farming and intensive animal agriculture often involve practices that compromise the

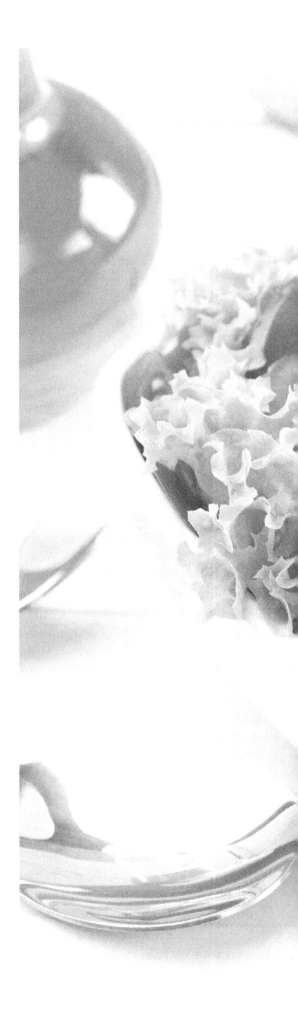

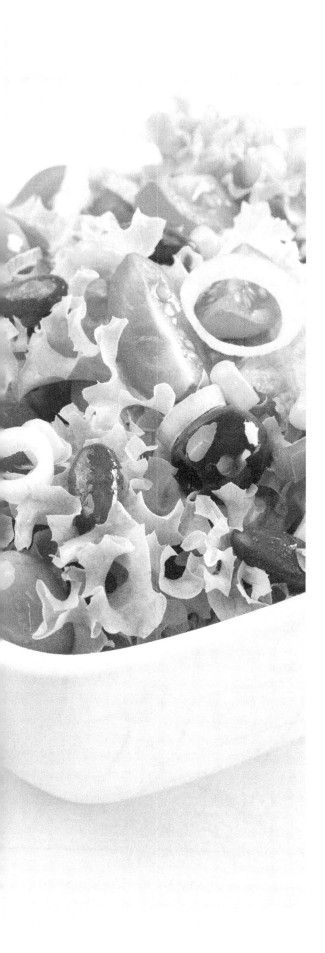

physical and psychological welfare of animals. By abstaining from animal products, individuals can express their opposition to these practices and promote a more compassionate approach towards animals.

Speciesism: Speciesism is the belief that humans have the right to exploit and use other animal species solely for their own benefit. Embracing a plant-based lifestyle challenges this notion and recognizes the inherent value and rights of all living beings, regardless of their species. It is a step towards rejecting the idea that animals exist solely for human use and consumption.

Sentience and Consciousness: Animals raised for food, particularly mammals and birds, possess the capacity to experience pain, pleasure, and a range of emotions. Many people believe that it is morally wrong to cause unnecessary harm or suffering to sentient beings. By choosing plant-based foods, individuals avoid contributing to the suffering and exploitation of animals for food.

Environmental Justice: The intensive animal agriculture industry often operates in ways that disproportionately impact marginalized communities and contribute to social injustices. Factory farms are frequently located in low-income areas, leading to environmental pollution, compromised health, and reduced quality of life for residents. A plant-based lifestyle supports environmental justice by reducing the demand for these industries and advocating for a more equitable and sustainable food system.

Global Food Security: The production of animal-based foods requires significant amounts of land, water, and resources. In a world with a growing population and increasing food demands, a shift towards plant-based diets can help address global food security challenges. By consuming plant-based foods, individuals contribute to a more efficient use of resources and enable greater access to nutritious food for all.

Cultural Sensitivity: Adopting a plant-based lifestyle while being mindful of cultural diversity is important. It's crucial to approach the topic with respect and understanding, acknowledging that cultural traditions, values, and dietary practices vary across different communities. Promoting plant-based options and engaging in dialogue can help bridge cultural gaps and encourage a more inclusive approach to ethical eating.

Personal Integrity and Consistency: Many individuals choose a plant-based lifestyle as an expression of their personal values and integrity. Aligning one's actions with their ethical beliefs is empowering and can contribute to a sense of coherence and authenticity in life. By living in accordance with one's values, individuals may experience a deeper sense of personal fulfillment and satisfaction.

Embracing a plant-based lifestyle involves reflecting on our relationship with animals, recognizing their inherent value, and making choices that minimize harm and promote compassion. It is a personal journey that requires empathy, mindfulness, and a commitment to ethical principles. By adopting a plant-based lifestyle, individuals can align their actions with their values and contribute to a more compassionate and just world for all living beings.

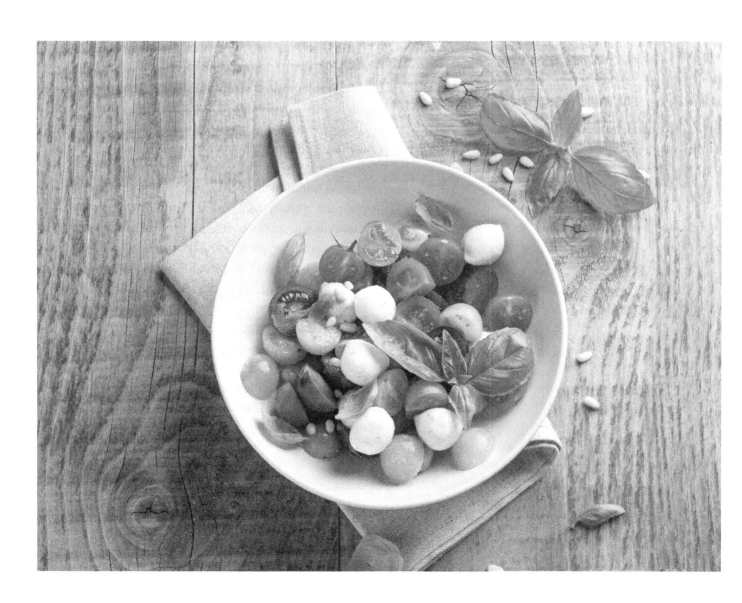

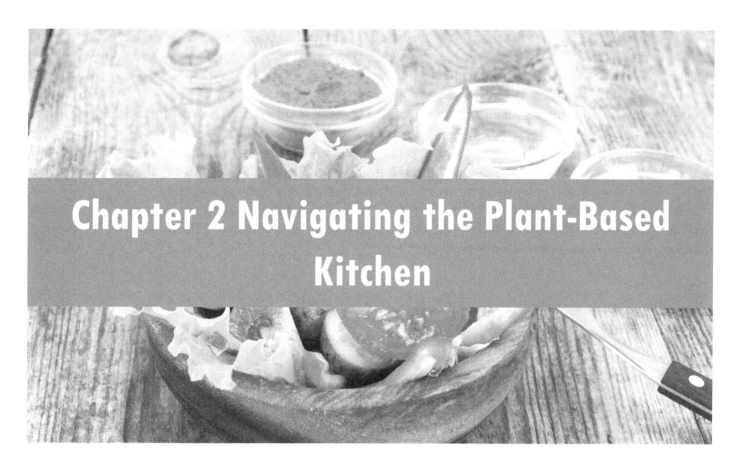

Chapter 2 Navigating the Plant-Based Kitchen

Essential Ingredients for a Plant-Based Pantry

Having a well-stocked plant-based pantry is essential for creating delicious and nutritious meals. Here are some essential ingredients to include in your plant-based pantry:

Whole Grains: Whole grains are a cornerstone of a plant-based diet, providing complex carbohydrates, fiber, and essential nutrients. Stock up on staples like brown rice, quinoa, oats, whole wheat pasta, and whole grain bread.

Legumes: Legumes, such as beans, lentils, and chickpeas, are excellent sources of protein, fiber, and various vitamins and minerals. Keep a variety of canned and dried legumes on hand for soups, stews, salads, and plant-based protein alternatives.

Nuts and Seeds: Nuts and seeds are versatile ingredients that add flavor, texture, and nutritional value to plant-based dishes. Keep a variety of options like almonds, walnuts, chia seeds, flaxseeds, and pumpkin seeds. They can be used in baking, smoothies, salads, and homemade nut butters.

Plant-Based Milk: Substitute dairy milk with plant-based alternatives like almond milk, soy milk, oat milk, or coconut milk. These options can be used in recipes, cereals, beverages, and as a creamer in coffee and tea.

Nutritional Yeast: Nutritional yeast is a popular ingredient among plant-based eaters. It adds a cheesy, nutty flavor to dishes and is a great source of vitamin B12. Use it as a topping for popcorn, pasta, or sprinkle it on roasted vegetables.

Healthy Oils: Keep a selection of healthy oils in your pantry, such as extra virgin olive oil, coconut oil, and avocado oil. These oils are suitable for cooking, sautéing, and dressing salads.

Spices and Herbs: Spices and herbs are essential for adding flavor to plant-based dishes. Have a variety of options like turmeric, cumin, paprika, garlic powder, oregano, basil, and parsley to enhance the taste of your meals.

Condiments and Sauces: Stock up on plant-based condiments and sauces to enhance the flavor of your dishes. Include items like soy sauce or tamari (gluten-free soy sauce), balsamic vinegar, tahini, hot sauce, mustard, and natural sweeteners like maple syrup or agave nectar.

Fresh and Frozen Fruits and Vegetables: While pantry staples are important, fresh and frozen fruits and vegetables are vital for a well-rounded plant-based diet. Ensure you have a variety of fresh produce, such as leafy greens, bell peppers, tomatoes, carrots, and berries. Frozen options are convenient for smoothies, stir-fries, and adding to recipes when fresh produce is not available.

Plant-Based Proteins: Incorporate plant-based protein sources like tofu, tempeh, and seitan into your pantry. These protein-rich options can be used in stir-fries, curries, sandwiches, and salads.

Remember to rotate your pantry items regularly to maintain freshness and check expiration dates. By keeping these essential ingredients in your plant-based pantry, you'll have a solid foundation for creating delicious and nutritious plant-based meals at home.

Tools and Equipment for Plant-Based Cooking

When it comes to plant-based cooking, having the right tools and equipment can make meal preparation easier and more enjoyable. Here are some essential tools and equipment for plant-based cooking:

High-Speed Blender: A high-speed blender is a versatile tool that can be used to make smoothies, sauces, soups, and even homemade nut butters. Look for a blender with a powerful motor and various speed settings to handle a wide range of ingredients.

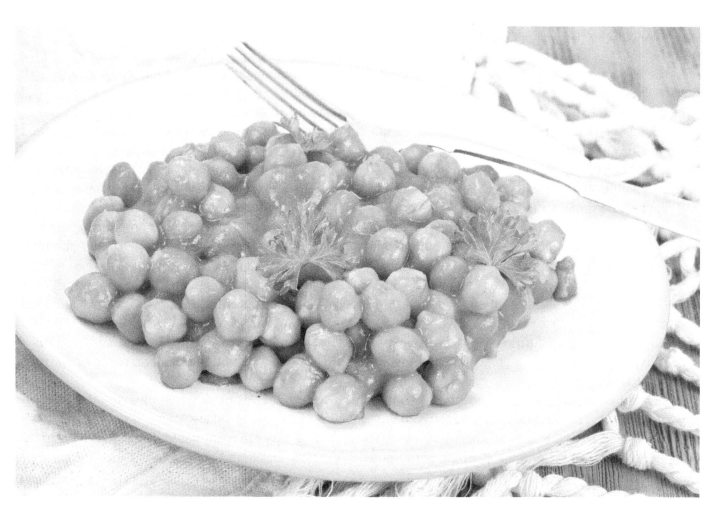

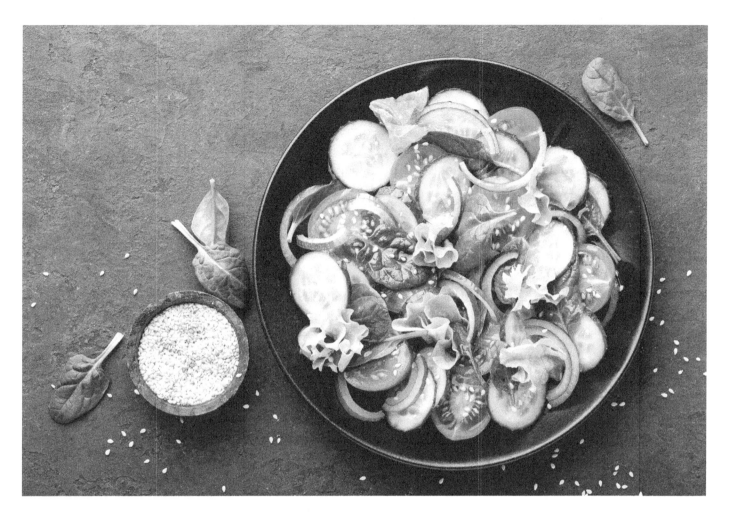

Food Processor: A food processor is handy for chopping, shredding, and blending ingredients. It's ideal for making homemade dips, spreads, energy balls, and even plant-based burger patties.

Chef's Knife and Cutting Board: A good-quality chef's knife and a sturdy cutting board are essential tools for any kitchen. Invest in a sharp, reliable knife that will make chopping fruits, vegetables, and herbs a breeze.

Vegetable Spiralizer: A vegetable spiralizer allows you to create noodles or "zoodles" from vegetables like zucchini, carrots, or sweet potatoes. It's a fun and healthy way to incorporate more vegetables into your meals.

Steamer Basket: A steamer basket is a fantastic tool for cooking vegetables while preserving their nutrients and natural flavors. It's perfect for steaming broccoli, cauliflower, Brussels sprouts, and other veggies.

Non-Stick Cookware: Non-stick cookware makes cooking plant-based meals a breeze, as it requires less oil and makes cleanup easier. Invest in a high-quality non-stick skillet, saucepan, and baking sheets for everyday cooking.

Oven or Air Fryer: An oven or air fryer is essential for baking, roasting, and crisping plant-based dishes. You can use it to roast vegetables, bake homemade bread, or even make oil-free crispy fries using an air fryer.

Slow Cooker or Instant Pot: A slow cooker or Instant Pot can be a time-saving tool for plant-based cooking. These appliances allow you to prepare hearty stews, soups, and bean dishes with minimal effort.

Salad Spinner: A salad spinner helps you wash and dry salad greens and other leafy vegetables efficiently. It's a must-have tool if you enjoy fresh salads regularly.

Mason Jars and Food Storage Containers: Mason jars and food storage containers are useful for storing prepped ingredients, homemade sauces, dressings, and leftovers. Opt for glass containers that are microwave-safe and have airtight lids.

Immersion Blender: An immersion blender, also known as a hand blender, is a convenient tool for blending soups, sauces, and smoothies directly in the pot or container. It's compact, easy to use, and requires less cleanup than a traditional blender.

Herb Grinder or Mortar and Pestle: If you enjoy using fresh herbs and spices in your plant-based dishes, having an herb grinder or mortar and pestle can help you grind them to release their flavors.

These are just a few of the essential tools and equipment for plant-based cooking. Depending on your preferences and the types of dishes you enjoy, you may find additional tools like a juicer, dehydrator, or pasta maker beneficial. Invest in high-quality tools that suit your cooking style and make your plant-based culinary adventures more efficient and enjoyable.

Fundamental Cooking Techniques for Plant-Based Meals

Mastering fundamental cooking techniques is essential for creating delicious and well-balanced plant-based meals. Here are some fundamental cooking techniques that will help you elevate your plant-based culinary skills:

Sautéing: Sautéing involves cooking ingredients in a small amount of oil or liquid over medium-high heat. It's a quick and versatile technique that works well for cooking vegetables, tofu, tempeh, and seitan. Sautéing helps develop flavors and adds a nice caramelization to the ingredients.

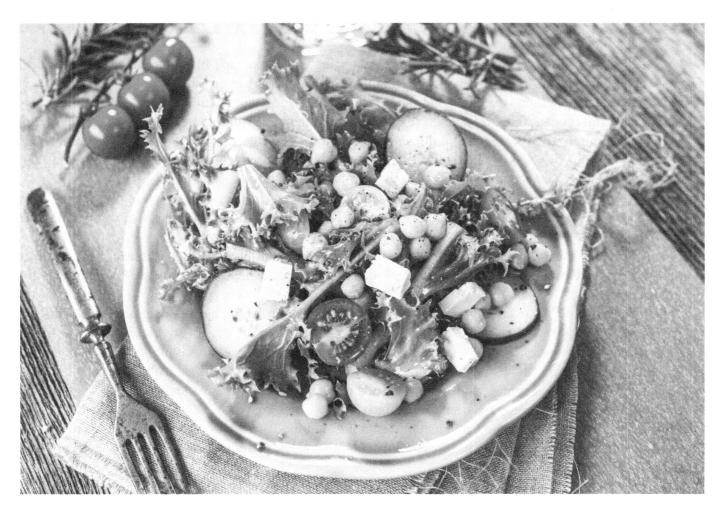

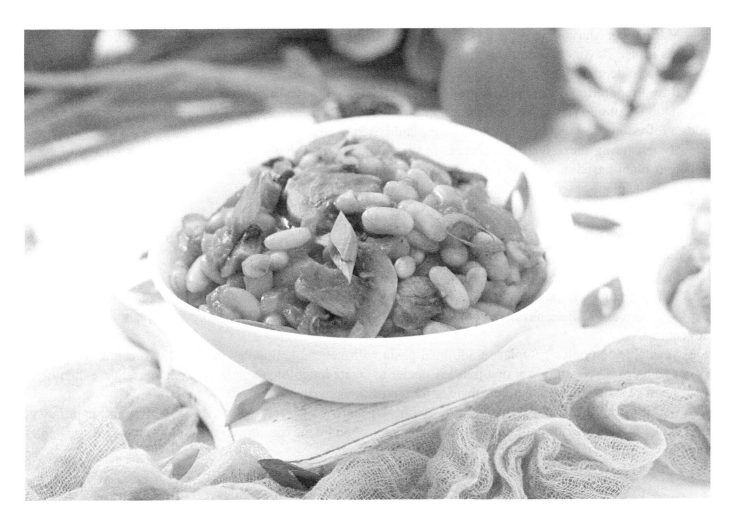

Roasting: Roasting is a dry heat cooking method that involves cooking ingredients in the oven at high temperatures. It's perfect for bringing out the natural sweetness and flavors of vegetables. Roasting vegetables like Brussels sprouts, carrots, cauliflower, and sweet potatoes creates a delicious caramelization and adds depth to your dishes.

Steaming: Steaming is a gentle cooking technique that helps retain the nutrients and natural flavors of ingredients. It involves cooking food over simmering water, either in a steamer basket or using a covered pot. Steaming is excellent for cooking vegetables, grains, and even tofu or dumplings.

Boiling: Boiling is a cooking technique that involves submerging ingredients in a liquid and cooking them at a high temperature. It's commonly used for cooking grains like rice, quinoa, and pasta. Boiling is also useful for blanching vegetables before using them in salads or stir-fries.

Stir-Frying: Stir-frying is a high-heat cooking technique that involves quickly cooking bite-sized pieces of ingredients in a small amount of oil in a wok or skillet. It's perfect for creating flavorful and vibrant plant-based stir-fries with an array of colorful vegetables, tofu, or tempeh.

Grilling: Grilling adds a smoky flavor and beautiful grill marks to ingredients. You can use a barbecue grill or a stovetop grill pan to grill vegetables, plant-based burgers, skewers, or even fruit. It's a fantastic technique for summer cookouts and adds depth to your plant-based dishes.

Blending: Blending is a technique that involves using a blender or food processor to create smooth textures and combine ingredients. It's perfect for making smoothies, sauces, soups, and creamy dressings. Blending helps create a velvety texture and combines flavors beautifully.

Baking: Baking is a versatile cooking technique that allows you to create a wide range of plant-based dishes, including bread, cakes, muffins, and even casseroles. It involves cooking food in an oven, surrounded by dry heat. Baking allows for delicious flavor development and texture transformations.

Marinating: Marinating is the process of soaking ingredients in a flavorful liquid mixture before cooking. It helps infuse flavors and tenderize ingredients. Marinating tofu, tempeh, or vegetables can enhance their taste and add depth to your plant-based dishes.

Raw Preparations: Raw preparations involve using ingredients in their natural, uncooked state. This technique is common in salads, smoothies, and raw desserts. It preserves the maximum nutrient content and adds a refreshing and vibrant element to your plant-based meals.

By mastering these fundamental cooking techniques, you'll have the skills to create a wide variety of delicious plant-based meals. Experiment with different ingredients, flavors, and cooking methods to discover your favorite plant-based dishes and expand your culinary repertoire.

Creative Plant-Based Cooking Techniques and Recipe Ideas

When it comes to plant-based cooking, there is no shortage of creative techniques and recipe ideas to explore. Here are some innovative cooking techniques and recipe ideas to inspire your plant-based culinary adventures:

Vegetable "Noodles": Replace traditional pasta with vegetable noodles made from zucchini, carrots, or sweet potatoes. Use a spiralizer or a julienne peeler to create long, thin strands of vegetables. Serve them with your favorite sauces or toss them in stir-fries for a nutritious twist.

Cauliflower Rice: Transform cauliflower into a grain-free alternative to rice. Simply pulse cauliflower florets in a food processor until they resemble rice grains. Sauté the cauliflower rice with spices and vegetables for a low-carb and nutrient-packed side dish.

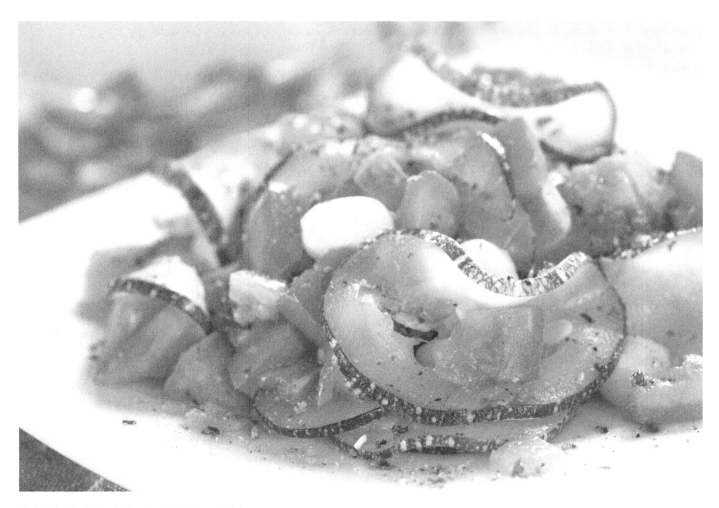

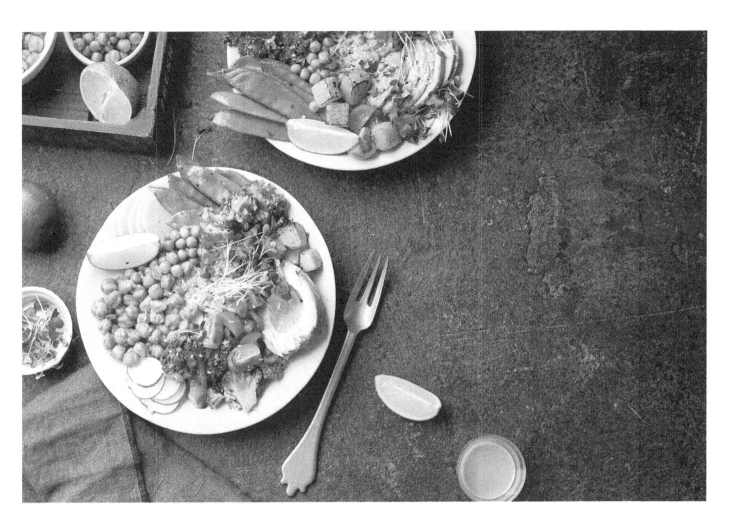

Stuffed Vegetables: Get creative by stuffing vegetables like bell peppers, zucchini, or portobello mushrooms with flavorful fillings. Consider using ingredients like quinoa, lentils, or a combination of sautéed vegetables, herbs, and spices. Bake or grill the stuffed vegetables until tender and delicious.

Veggie Burgers and Meatballs: Experiment with homemade veggie burger or meatball recipes using plant-based ingredients like black beans, chickpeas, lentils, mushrooms, or tofu. Combine them with herbs, spices, breadcrumbs, and binding agents to create flavorful and satisfying plant-based alternatives.

Raw Desserts: Explore the world of raw desserts that are made without baking or cooking. Create delectable treats like raw vegan cheesecakes, energy balls, or chocolate mousse using nuts, dates, coconut oil, and cacao powder. These desserts are rich in flavor and packed with nutrient-dense ingredients.

Fermentation: Embrace the art of fermentation by making your own plant-based fermented foods. Try making sauerkraut, kimchi, or fermented cashew cheese. Fermented foods are not only delicious but also promote gut health and provide beneficial probiotics.

Smoked or Grilled Vegetables: Experiment with smoking or grilling vegetables to add a smoky flavor and depth to your dishes. Use a smoker or grill to infuse flavors into vegetables like eggplant, bell peppers, or corn. Serve them as a side dish or use them as a filling in wraps and sandwiches.

Plant-Based Cheese Making: Dive into the world of plant-based cheese making using nuts like cashews or almonds. Soak the nuts, blend them with probiotics or yeast, and allow them to ferment and develop complex flavors. With some creativity and patience, you can create an array of dairy-free cheeses.

Aquafaba: Explore the wonders of aquafaba, the liquid from cooked chickpeas or the liquid found in canned chickpeas. It can be whipped into a fluffy foam to replace egg whites in recipes or used as a binder in baked goods.

Vegan Ice Cream: Experiment with making your own vegan ice cream using frozen bananas as the base. Blend frozen bananas with other fruits, nut butters, or cacao powder to create a creamy and dairy-free frozen treat.

These are just a few creative plant-based cooking techniques and recipe ideas to get you started. Don't be afraid to explore, experiment, and adapt recipes to suit your taste preferences and dietary needs. With a bit of creativity and an open mind, you can create a wide variety of delicious and innovative plant-based dishes that will impress both vegans and non-vegans alike.

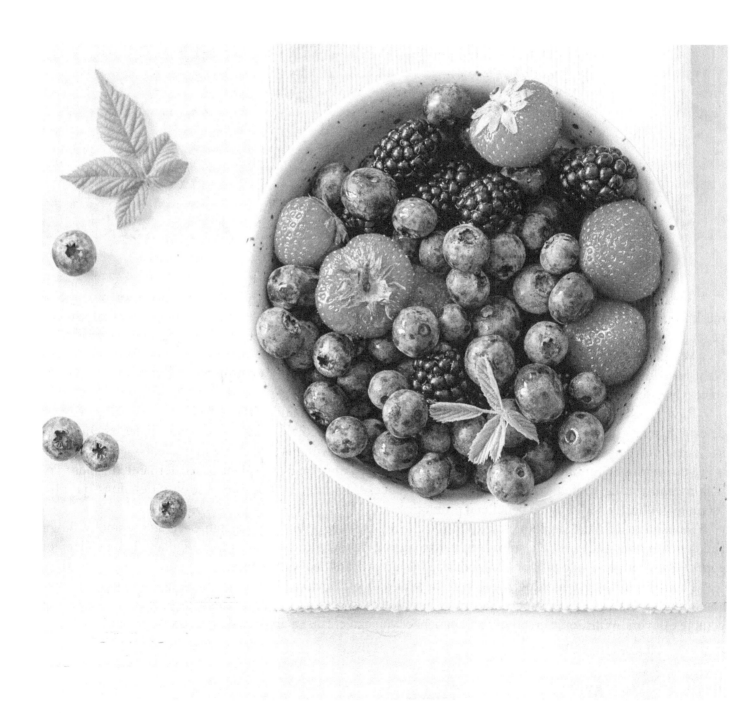

30 Days Plant-Based Diet Meal Plan

DAYS	BREAKFAST	LUNCH	DINNER	SNACK/DESSERT
1	Savory Oatmeal	Fluffy Mashed Potatoes with Gravy	Greek Salad in a Jar	Quinoa Banana Muffins
2	To the Power of Four Overnight Oats	Ratatouille	Pepperoncini Lentil Crunch Salad	Chocolate Chip Oat Cookies
3	Spelt Berry Hot Breakfast Cereal	Tangy Cabbage, Apples, and Potatoes	Lentil Salad with Lemon and Fresh Herbs	Gluten-Free Vegan Muffins
4	Sweet Potato Pie Oatmeal	Aloo Gobi (Potato and Cauliflower Curry)	Caramelized Onion Potato Salad	Caramel-Coconut Frosted Brownies
5	Whole-Wheat Blueberry Muffins	Millet-Stuffed Portobello Mushrooms	Zingy Melon and Mango Salad	Two-Ingredient Peanut Butter Fudge
6	Blueberry, Cinnamon, and Pecan French Toast	Lemony Steamed Kale with Olives	Chickpea Apple Salad	Almond Truffles with Toasted Coconut
7	Chocolate Cherry Oats Bowl	Summer Squash and Blossom Sauté with Mint and Peas	Tomato, Corn and Bean Salad	Nice Cream
8	Savory Ginger Green Onion Crepes	Roasted Veggies with Tofu	Pineapple Quinoa Salad	Gluten-Free Vegan Waffles
9	Banana-Date Shake with Oats	Spicy Carrots with Coriander	Broccoli Caesar with Smoky Tempeh Bits	Cacao Pudding
10	Strawberries and Cream Overnight Oatmeal	Loaded Frijoles	Pinto Salsa Bowl	Peanut Butter Nice Cream
11	Overnight Chocolate Chia Pudding	Chickpea of the Sea Salad	Smoky Potato Salad over Greens	Peanut Butter Cookies
12	Buckwheat Protein Bread	Baked Spaghetti Squash with Spicy Lentil Sauce	Creamy Fruit Salad	Tropical Colada Frozen Pops
13	Peaches and Cream Overnight Oats	Blackened Sprouts	Ancient Grains Salad	Homemade Applesauce with Raisins and Nuts
14	Cookies for Breakfast	Indian Spiced Eggplant	Go-To Kale Salad with "Master Cleanse" Dressing	Nutty Raspberry Thumbprint Cookies
15	Spinach Crepes	Glowing, Fermented Vegetable Tangle	Creamy Potato Salad	Vanilla Corn Cake with Roasted Strawberries
16	Sunshine Muffins	Fennel and Green Cabbage Kraut	Slaw Salad and Avocado Dressing	Sweet Potato Spice Cake
17	Spiced Pumpkin Muffins	Stir-Fried Vegetables with Miso and Sake	Wedge Salad with Avocado Citrus Dressing	Almond-Date Energy Bites
18	Simple Tofu Scramble	Grilled Eggplant "Steaks"	Apple Broccoli Crunch Bowl	Coconut Chia Pudding

DAYS	BREAKFAST	LUNCH	DINNER	SNACK/DESSERT
19	Red Flannel Beet Hash with Dill	Tangy Cabbage and Kale Slaw	Chickpea Salad with Vegetables	Whole Wheat Berry Muffins
20	Sweet Potato and Black Bean Hash	Savory Slow Cooker Stuffing	Quinoa Arugula Salad	Pumpkin Bread Pudding
21	Applesauce Crumble Muffins	Sautéed Collard Greens	Purple Potato and Kale Salad	Homemade Caramel with Dates and Peanut Butter
22	Zucchini Bread Oatmeal	Vegetable Korma Curry	Roasted Root Vegetable Salad Bowl	Sweet Potato and Chocolate Pudding
23	Banana Almond Granola	Gingered Brussels Sprout and Shiitake Pot Stickers	Curried Kale Slaw	Coconut and Tahini Bliss Balls
24	Mango, Pineapple, and Spinach Smoothie	Baked Spaghetti Squash with Swiss Chard	Blueprint: Classic Kale Salad	Banana Bread Scones
25	Green Banana Smoothie	Braised Red Cabbage with Beans	Chicken and Mixed Greens Salad	Poached Pears
26	Fruit Salad	Shaved Fennel and Lemon Pickle	Vegan "Toona" Salad	Zabaglione Cashew Cream
27	Seeds, Nuts, and Fruit Baked Granola	Sweet Potato Tacos	Crunchy Curry Salad	Walnut Brownies
28	Overnight Pumpkin Spice Chia Pudding	Baked Falafel	Taco Tempeh Salad	Gooey Bittersweet Chocolate Pudding Cake
29	Best Whole Wheat Pancakes	Mac 'N' Mince	Mango Black Bean Salad	Pistachio Protein Ice Cream
30	Cherry Pecan Granola Bars	Chickpea Pâté	Spinach Salad with Sweet Smoky Dressing	Salted Caramel Bites

Chapter 3 Breakfasts

Savory Oatmeal

Prep time: 10 minutes | Cook time: 10 minutes | Makes 2 bowls

1 cup gluten-free old-fashioned rolled oats	yeast
1 carrot, peeled and shredded	½ chopped avocado
1½ cups water	2 tablespoons roasted pumpkin seeds
1 cup stemmed and chopped kale	Smoked paprika or crushed red pepper (optional)
¼ cup salsa or marinara sauce	Salt and black pepper (optional)
2 tablespoons nutritional	

1. In a small saucepan over medium heat, combine the oats and carrot. Add the desired amount of water to achieve your preferred oatmeal consistency (around 1½ cups water for thicker oatmeal). 2. Bring the mixture to a simmer and cook, stirring often, until the oats and carrot are tender, approximately 5 minutes. 3. Stir in the kale, salsa, and nutritional yeast. 4. Transfer the oatmeal to a bowl and top with avocado and pumpkin seeds. Add smoked paprika and crushed red pepper for extra flavor if desired. Season with salt and pepper to taste, and serve your delicious Savory Oatmeal! Enjoy this hearty and nutritious dish!

Per Serving: (½ bowl)

calories: 153 | fat: 7g | protein: 9g | carbs: 24g | fiber: 7g

To the Power of Four Overnight Oats

Prep time: 10 minutes | Cook time: 0 minutes | Serves 2

3½ cups unsweetened almond milk	¼ cup sunflower seed kernels
2 cups old-fashioned oats	4 tablespoons peanut butter, divided
¼ cup maple syrup (optional)	
2 tablespoons chia seeds	Sunflower seed kernels, for garnish (optional)
2 tablespoons unsweetened shredded coconut	

1. In a large bowl, combine all the ingredients except for 2 tablespoons of peanut butter and sunflower seeds. Mix well; the mixture may seem wet initially, but the chia seeds and oats will absorb some of the milk overnight. Cover the bowl and refrigerate to set overnight. 2. In the morning, take two bowls and spread the remaining 2 tablespoons of peanut butter around the inside of each bowl. Fill each bowl with the overnight oats mixture. Garnish with sunflower seeds if desired. Enjoy your delicious and nutritious To the Power of Four Overnight Oats!

Per Serving:

calories: 559 | fat: 21g | protein: 24g | carbs: 46g | fiber: 10g

Blueberry, Cinnamon, and Pecan French Toast

Prep time: 10 minutes | Cook time: 2 to 3 hours | Serves 4 to 6

2 tablespoons ground flaxseed	1 teaspoon ground cinnamon
5 tablespoons water	1 tablespoon vanilla extract
1 (16-ounce / 454-g) loaf crusty whole-grain bread	Nonstick cooking spray (optional)
1 overripe banana, peeled	2 cups fresh or frozen blueberries, divided
1 (14½-ounce / 411-g) can full-fat coconut milk	¼ cup chopped pecans, for serving
1 cup unsweetened plant-based milk	Maple syrup, for serving (optional)
1 tablespoon chia seeds	

1. Prepare flax eggs by mixing flaxseed and water in a small bowl. Let it rest while you continue. 2. Slice bread into 1- to 2-inch chunks and place them in a large casserole dish. 3. In a blender, combine banana, coconut milk, plant-based milk, chia seeds, cinnamon, vanilla, and flax eggs. Blend until well combined, then pour the mixture over the bread. Cover and refrigerate for at least 30 minutes to let the bread soak up the custard. 4. Grease the slow cooker with cooking spray or use a slow cooker liner. Layer half of the bread and custard mixture in the slow cooker, add 1 cup of blueberries, then repeat with the remaining mixture and another cup of blueberries. 5. Cover and cook on High for 2 to 3 hours or on Low for 4 to 5 hours. 6. To serve, top each portion with a tablespoon of pecans and drizzle with maple syrup if desired. Enjoy your delicious Blueberry, Cinnamon, and Pecan French Toast!

Per Serving:

calories: 644 | fat: 31g | protein: 5g | carbs: 81g | fiber: 18g

Simple Tofu Scramble

Prep time: 5 minutes | Cook time: 15 minutes | Serves 2 to 4

2 tablespoons red miso paste	yeast
½ cup water	1 teaspoon dried parsley
2 (14-ounce / 397-g)	½ teaspoon garlic powder
packages firm tofu, drained	¼ teaspoon ground turmeric
2 tablespoons onion powder	¼ teaspoon freshly ground
2 tablespoons nutritional	black pepper

1. In a sauté pan or skillet, dissolve miso in water. 2. Loosely crumble tofu into the miso-water mixture. 3. Stir in onion powder, nutritional yeast, parsley, garlic powder, turmeric, and pepper. Cook over medium heat, stirring occasionally, for 10 to 15 minutes, or until heated through and most of the liquid is absorbed. Remove from the heat and enjoy your delicious Tofu Scramble!

Per Serving:

calories: 84 | fat: 2g | protein: 7g | carbs: 9g | fiber: 0g

Red Flannel Beet Hash with Dill

Prep time: 15 minutes | Cook time: 55 minutes | Serves 6

2 medium Yukon gold	diced
potatoes, chopped into	1 teaspoon ground coriander
1-inch pieces	Salt and pepper, to taste
2 medium beets, peeled and	(optional)
chopped into ½-inch pieces	2 green onions, thinly sliced
1 tablespoon apple cider	¼ cup lightly packed
vinegar	chopped fresh dill
2 tablespoons virgin olive oil	½ ripe avocado, peeled,
(optional)	pitted and chopped
1 medium cooking onion,	

1. In a large saucepan or braiser-style pot, place chopped potatoes and beets. Cover the vegetables with cold water by 1 inch and add apple cider vinegar. Bring to a boil, then simmer until potatoes are tender and beets are just tender, about 20 minutes. Drain the vegetables and set aside. 2. Heat olive oil in a large skillet over medium heat. Add onions and cook until lightly soft, about 3 minutes. Add coriander, salt (if using), and pepper, stirring until fragrant, about 30 seconds. 3. Add the drained potatoes and beets to the skillet, spreading them out in a single layer. Let sit for 5 minutes before stirring. Flip and stir the hash every 5 minutes, cooking for an additional 20 minutes or until the edges of the potatoes begin to crisp. 4. Lightly toss the hash with green onions and dill. Serve the hash hot, and top with chopped avocado. Enjoy your delicious Red Flannel Beet Hash with Dill!

Per Serving:

calories: 144 | fat: 7g | protein: 3g | carbs: 19g | fiber: 4g

Green Banana Smoothie

Prep time: 5 minutes | Cook time: 0 minutes | Makes 2 glasses

2½ to 3 sliced frozen	stems removed
bananas	1½ cups plant-based milk
1½ cups spinach or kale,	

1. simply blend all the ingredients on high in a blender until smooth. Enjoy your refreshing and nutritious drink!

Per Serving: (1 glass)

calories: 134 | fat: 4g | protein: 8g | carbs: 16g | fiber: 3g

Mango, Pineapple, and Spinach Smoothie

Prep time: 5 minutes | Cook time: 0 minutes | Serves 1

1¼ cups unsweetened vanilla	⅓ cup pineapple chunks
coconut milk (or other	⅓ cup mango chunks
unsweetened milk substitute)	¼ cup almond flour
1 small avocado, peeled and	1 teaspoon maple syrup
pitted	(optional)
1 cup fresh spinach	3 ice cubes

1. Place milk, avocado, spinach, pineapple, mango, flour, maple syrup (if using), and ice cubes in a blender. 2. Blend on high until smooth or desired consistency is reached. 3. Pour the smoothie into a glass and enjoy your refreshing and nutritious drink!

Per Serving:

calories: 604 | fat: 42g | protein: 17g | carbs: 52g | fiber: 19g

Fruit Salad

Prep time: 15 minutes | Cook time: 0 minutes | Serves 4

1 pint fresh strawberries,	2 tablespoons fresh lemon
stems removed, sliced	juice
1 pint fresh blueberries	2 tablespoons date syrup
2 cups seedless grapes	(optional)
1 ripe pear, cored and diced	Pinch ground cinnamon

1. Combine all ingredients in a bowl and mix well. Chill until ready to serve.

Per Serving:

calories: 172 | fat: 0g | protein: 1g | carbs: 44g | fiber: 5g

Sweet Potato and Black Bean Hash

Prep time: 10 minutes | Cook time: 2 to 3 hours | Serves 4 to 6

1 shallot, diced	rinsed
2 cups peeled, chopped	1 teaspoon paprika
sweet potatoes (about 1 large	½ teaspoon onion powder
or 2 small)	½ teaspoon garlic powder
1 medium bell pepper (any	¼ cup store-bought low-
color), diced	sodium vegetable broth
2 garlic cloves, minced	4 to 6 tablespoons
1 (14½-ounce / 411-g) can	unsweetened plant-based
black beans, drained and	milk

1. Place shallot, sweet potatoes, bell pepper, garlic, black beans, paprika, onion powder, garlic powder, and broth in the slow cooker. Stir to combine. Cover and cook on Low for 2 to 3 hours until sweet potatoes are soft. 2. Remove the lid and add milk, starting with 4 tablespoons, stirring to create a creamy sauce. Add more milk as needed and let it heat through for a few minutes before serving. Enjoy your delicious and creamy Sweet Potato and Black Bean Hash!

Per Serving:

calories: 251 | fat: 1g | protein: 9g | carbs: 53g | fiber: 14g

Applesauce Crumble Muffins

Prep time: 10 minutes | Cook time: 15 to 20 minutes | Makes 12 muffins

1 teaspoon coconut oil,	1 teaspoon pure vanilla
for greasing muffin tins	extract
(optional)	2 cups whole-grain flour
2 tablespoons nut butter or	1 teaspoon baking soda
seed butter	½ teaspoon baking powder
1½ cups unsweetened	1 teaspoon ground cinnamon
applesauce	Pinch sea salt (optional)
⅓ cup coconut sugar	½ cup walnuts, chopped
(optional)	Toppings (optional):
½ cup nondairy milk	¼ cup walnuts
2 tablespoons ground	¼ cup coconut sugar
flaxseed	(optional)
1 teaspoon apple cider	½ teaspoon ground
vinegar	cinnamon

1. Preheat the oven to 350ºF (180ºC) and prepare two 6-cup muffin tins with coconut oil or muffin cups. 2. Mix nut butter, applesauce, coconut sugar (if using), milk, flaxseed, vinegar, and vanilla until combined. 3. In a separate bowl, sift together flour, baking soda, baking powder, cinnamon, salt (if using), and chopped walnuts. 4. Combine wet and dry ingredients until just mixed. 5. Spoon ¼ cup batter into each muffin cup and add optional toppings. Bake for 15 to 20 minutes or until a toothpick comes out clean. Enjoy moist and delicious Applesauce Crumble Muffins!

Per Serving: (1 muffin)

calories: 178 | fat: 6g | protein: 4g | carbs: 28g | fiber: 3g

Zucchini Bread Oatmeal

Prep time: 5 minutes | Cook time: 20 minutes | Serves 4

2 cups rolled oats	½ cup raisins
1 medium zucchini, grated	1 tablespoon maple syrup
4 cups water	(optional)
½ cup unsweetened plant-	Pinch of salt (optional)
based milk	2 medium bananas, sliced
1 tablespoon ground	4 tablespoons chopped
cinnamon	walnuts (optional)

1. In a medium saucepan over medium-high heat, combine oats, zucchini, and water. Bring to a boil, then lower the heat to medium-low and simmer, stirring often, for about 15 minutes until the oats are soft and creamy. Remove from heat and add plant-based milk, cinnamon, raisins, maple syrup, and salt (if using). Stir well. 2. Divide the oatmeal into 4 bowls and top each portion with half of a sliced banana and 1 tablespoon of walnuts (if using). Enjoy your delicious Zucchini Bread Oatmeal!

Per Serving:

calories: 301 | fat: 4g | protein: 9g | carbs: 62g | fiber: 8g

Banana Almond Granola

Prep time: 10 minutes | Cook time: 50 minutes | Serves 16

8 cups rolled oats	1 teaspoon almond extract
2 cups pitted and chopped	1 teaspoon salt, or to taste
dates	(optional)
2 ripe bananas, peeled and	1 cup slivered almonds,
chopped	toasted (optional)

1. Preheat the oven to 275ºF (135ºC) and line two baking pans with parchment paper. 2. In a large mixing bowl, combine oats. 3. In a saucepan, cook dates with water until soft, then blend with bananas, almond extract, and salt until smooth. 4. Add the date mixture to the oats and mix well. 5. Spread the mixture evenly on the prepared pans. 6. Bake for 40 to 50 minutes, stirring every 10 minutes, until crispy. 7. Let the granola cool and add slivered almonds if desired. Store in an airtight container for later enjoyment.

Per Serving:

calories: 220 | fat: 6g | protein: 10g | carbs: 49g | fiber: 10g

Crazy Quinoa Protein Muffins

Prep time: 15 minutes | Cook time: 35 minutes | Serves 6

½ cup quinoa
2 tablespoons ground chia seeds
¼ cup almond flour
3 tablespoons vanilla protein powder
½ teaspoon salt (optional)
½ cup dates, chopped small

2 tablespoons coconut oil (optional)
3 tablespoons maple syrup (optional)
1 teaspoon vanilla extract
¼ cup unsweetened shredded coconut
½ cup raisins

1. Rinse the quinoa and place in a small saucepan with a lid. Cover with ½ cup water and bring to a boil over medium-high heat. Cover and turn down to low. Let cook for 20 minutes and then remove from the heat. Take off the lid and let cool. 2. Preheat the oven to 450ºF (235ºC). Line six muffin cups with paper liners. 3. Mix the ground chia seeds with ¼ cup plus 2 tablespoons water and set aside. 4. Add the almond flour, protein powder, and salt (if desired) to a small bowl. Mix well. Add the dates and mix to coat. Set aside. 5. Put the coconut oil (if desired) in a medium bowl. If it is not liquid already, put in the microwave and heat for 10 to 20 seconds or until melted. Remove from microwave and add the maple syrup, if desired. Stir well. When cool, add the chia seed mixture, vanilla extract, coconut, almond flour mixture, cooked quinoa, and raisins. Mix well. 6. Divide the batter between the six muffin cups and bake 12 to 15 minutes, until a toothpick inserted in the center comes out clean.

Per Serving: (1 muffin)

calories: 179 | fat: 6g | protein: 7g | carbs: 26g | fiber: 5g

Fruited Barley

Prep time: 10 minutes | Cook time: 55 minutes | Serves 2

1 to 1½ cups orange juice
1 cup pearled barley
2 tablespoons dried currants
3 to 4 dried unsulfured apricots, chopped

1 small cinnamon stick
⅛ teaspoon ground cloves
Pinch salt, or to taste (optional)

1. Bring 1 cup of water and 1 cup of the orange juice to a boil in a medium saucepan over medium heat. Add the barley, currants, apricots, cinnamon stick, cloves, and salt, if using. Bring the mixture to a boil, cover, reduce the heat to medium-low, and cook for 45 minutes. If the barley is not tender after 45 minutes, add up to an additional ½ cup of orange juice and cook for another 10 minutes. 2. Remove the cinnamon stick before serving.

Per Serving:

calories: 420 | fat: 1g | protein: 10g | carbs: 93g | fiber: 16g

Cookies for Breakfast

Prep time: 10 minutes | Cook time: 20 minutes | Makes 12 cookies

1¼ cups certified gluten-free rolled oats
1 teaspoon ground cinnamon
½ teaspoon baking soda
½ teaspoon fine sea salt (optional)
½ cup almond flour
¼ cup brown rice flour
½ cup mashed ripe banana
½ cup smooth almond butter,

stirred
3 tablespoons pure maple syrup (optional)
2 tablespoons ground flaxseed
3 tablespoons liquid virgin coconut oil (optional)
1 teaspoon pure vanilla extract

1. Preheat the oven to 350ºF (180ºC) and line a baking sheet with parchment paper. 2. In a large bowl, mix rolled oats, cinnamon, baking soda, sea salt (if using), almond flour, and brown rice flour. 3. In a food processor, blend mashed banana, almond butter, maple syrup (if using), ground flaxseed, and coconut oil (if using) until smooth. 4. Combine the almond butter mixture with the dry ingredients until you have a stiff cookie dough. 5. Drop 2 tablespoons of dough per cookie onto the baking sheet and flatten each mound. 6. Bake for 15 to 17 minutes until lightly golden brown. Let the cookies cool completely before storing in an airtight container. Enjoy them for up to 5 days on the counter or freeze them individually for later.

Per Serving:

calories: 160 | fat: 10g | protein: 5g | carbs: 17g | fiber: 4g

Spelt Berry Hot Breakfast Cereal

Prep time: 5 minutes | Cook time: 55 minutes | Serves 2

1 cup spelt berries
¼ teaspoon salt (optional)
⅛ teaspoon ground cinnamon
⅛ teaspoon ground cloves

2 cups unsweetened almond milk
¾ cup dates, pitted and chopped
¼ teaspoon orange zest

1. In a medium saucepan, bring 2½ cups of water to a boil. Add the spelt, salt (if desired), cinnamon, and cloves. Cover the pot and let the mixture come to a boil. Reduce the heat to medium-low and cook for 45 to 50 minutes until the spelt is tender. Drain any excess water. 2. Stir in the almond milk, dates, and orange zest to the cooked spelt berries. Simmer the mixture over medium-low heat for 10 to 12 minutes, until it becomes creamy and heated through. Enjoy your comforting and nutritious Spelt Berry Hot Breakfast Cereal!

Per Serving:

calories: 423 | fat: 2g | protein: 18g | carbs: 88g | fiber: 13g

Buckwheat Protein Bread

Prep time: 15 minutes | Cook time: 40 minutes | Serves 6

1 cup buckwheat flour	¼ cup raisins
½ cup pea protein	3-inch piece ginger, minced
¼ cup chia seeds	2 cups water

1. Preheat your oven to 375ºF (190ºC) and line a small loaf pan with parchment paper. 2. Using a food processor, blend all the ingredients except the raisins until you get a smooth and sticky dough. Alternatively, mix all the ingredients in a large bowl using a handheld mixer. 3. Stir in the raisins to distribute them evenly in the dough. 4. Transfer the dough to the prepared loaf pan, spreading it evenly and smoothing the top with a tablespoon. 5. Bake the bread in the preheated oven for 40 minutes. 6. Once baked, let the bread cool completely to prevent it from falling apart when sliced. 7. Store the Buckwheat Protein Bread in an airtight container and enjoy it within 4 days. You can also freeze it for up to 90 days and thaw at room temperature when needed. Enjoy your nutritious and delicious bread!

Per Serving:

calories: 376 | fat: 30g | protein: 16g | carbs: 11g | fiber: 9g

Sunshine Muffins

Prep time: 15 minutes | Cook time: 30 minutes | Makes 6 muffins

1 teaspoon coconut oil, for greasing muffin tins (optional)	cinnamon
	½ teaspoon ground ginger (optional)
2 tablespoons almond butter or sunflower seed butter	¼ teaspoon ground nutmeg (optional)
¼ cup nondairy milk	¼ teaspoon allspice (optional)
1 orange, peeled	¾ cup rolled oats or whole-grain flour
1 carrot, coarsely chopped	
2 tablespoons chopped dried apricots or other dried fruit	1 teaspoon baking powder
	½ teaspoon baking soda
3 tablespoons molasses	Mix-Ins (optional):
2 tablespoons ground flaxseed	½ cup rolled oats
1 teaspoon apple cider vinegar	2 tablespoons raisins or other chopped dried fruit
1 teaspoon pure vanilla extract	2 tablespoons sunflower seeds
½ teaspoon ground	

1. Preheat the oven to 350ºF (180ºC) and prepare a 6-cup muffin tin with coconut oil or muffin cups. 2. In a food processor or blender, purée nut butter, milk, orange, carrot, apricots, molasses, flaxseed, vinegar, vanilla, cinnamon, ginger, nutmeg, and allspice until somewhat smooth. 3. Grind oats to flour consistency and mix with baking powder and baking soda in a large bowl. 4. Combine wet ingredients with dry ingredients until just combined. Fold in mix-ins if desired. 5. Spoon about ¼ cup batter into each muffin cup and bake for 30 minutes or until a toothpick inserted in the center comes out clean. Adjust baking time as needed for moisture content. Enjoy your Sunshine Muffins!

Per Serving: (1 muffin)

calories: 226 | fat: 8g | protein: 7g | carbs: 34g | fiber: 6g

Overnight Chocolate Chia Pudding

Prep time: 2 minutes | Cook time: 0 minutes | Serves 2

¼ cup chia seeds	powder
1 cup unsweetened nondairy milk	1 teaspoon vanilla extract
	1 teaspoon pure maple syrup (optional)
2 tablespoons raw cacao	

1. In a large bowl, stir together the chia seeds, milk, cacao powder, vanilla, and maple syrup (if using). 2. Divide the mixture between 2 (½-pint) covered glass jars or containers. 3. Refrigerate the jars overnight. 4. Before serving, give the pudding a good stir to combine the ingredients. Enjoy your delicious and nutritious chocolate chia pudding!

Per Serving: (1 jar)

calories: 213 | fat: 10g | protein: 9g | carbs: 20g | fiber: 15g

Spinach Crepes

Prep time: 5 minutes | Cook time: 10 minutes | Makes 2 crepes

½ cup chickpea flour	ground black pepper, to taste (optional)
1 teaspoon ground flaxseeds	
¾ cup water	1 teaspoon coconut oil, divided, for frying (optional)
2 handfuls of spinach	
Celtic sea salt and freshly	

Your choice of fillings—our personal favorites are sautéed mushrooms, bell peppers, cherry tomatoes, fresh herbs, and avocado

1. In a blender, combine chickpea flour, flaxseeds, water, spinach, salt (if using), and pepper until well combined. Let the batter rest for 5 to 10 minutes. 2. Heat ½ teaspoon coconut oil (if using) in a 7-inch skillet over medium heat. Pour ¼ cup of the batter into the pan and swirl to form an even crepe. 3. Cook for about 2 minutes or until bubbles appear on the crepe's surface, then flip and cook the other side for 30 seconds to 1 minute. 4. Remove the crepe from the pan, place on a plate, and cover with a cloth to keep warm. 5. Repeat with the remaining oil and batter. 6. Fill the crepes with your desired fillings. Enjoy your delicious Spinach Crepes!

Per Serving:

calories: 138 | fat: 5g | protein: 8g | carbs: 17g | fiber: 5g

Savory Ginger Green Onion Crepes

Prep time: 5 minutes | Cook time: 20 minutes | Makes 8 crepes

⅔ cup chickpea flour	1 piece of fresh ginger,
⅔ cup buckwheat flour	peeled and finely grated
2 green onions, finely sliced	1 tablespoon sesame seeds
2 teaspoons fine sea salt	1½ cups filtered water
(optional)	Olive oil spray, for cooking
1 teaspoon chili powder	(optional)

1. Preheat the oven to 275°F (135°C) with a baking sheet inside. 2. In a large bowl, combine chickpea flour, buckwheat flour, sliced green onions, sea salt (optional), chili powder, grated ginger, and sesame seeds. Whisk together. 3. Add filtered water to the flour mixture and whisk until a thin crepe batter forms. Let it rest for 30 minutes. 4. Heat a crepe pan over medium-high heat. Add batter and spread it thinly. Cook each crepe until dry and lightly browned on both sides. Keep cooked crepes warm in the oven while making the rest. Enjoy your delicious Savory Ginger Green Onion Crepes!

Per Serving: (1 crepe)

calories: 87 | fat: 2g | protein: 4g | carbs: 14g | fiber: 3g

Spiced Pumpkin Muffins

Prep time: 15 minutes | Cook time: 20 minutes | Makes 12 muffins

2 tablespoons ground	⅛ teaspoon ground cloves
flaxseed	1 cup pumpkin purée
¼ cup water	½ cup pure maple syrup
1¾ cups whole wheat flour	(optional)
2 teaspoons baking powder	¼ cup unsweetened
1½ teaspoons ground	applesauce
cinnamon	¼ cup unsweetened nondairy
½ teaspoon baking soda	milk
½ teaspoon ground ginger	1½ teaspoons vanilla extract
¼ teaspoon ground nutmeg	

1. Preheat the oven to 350°F (180°C) and line a 12-cup metal muffin pan with parchment-paper liners or use a silicone muffin pan. 2. In a small bowl, whisk together flaxseed and water, then set aside. 3. In a large bowl, whisk together flour, baking powder, cinnamon, baking soda, ginger, nutmeg, and cloves. 4. In a medium bowl, stir together pumpkin purée, maple syrup (if using), applesauce, milk, and vanilla. Fold the wet ingredients into the dry ingredients using a spatula. 5. Gently fold in the soaked flaxseed until evenly combined, being careful not to overmix the batter. Spoon about ¼ cup of batter per muffin into the prepared muffin pan. 6. Bake for 18 to 20 minutes, or until a toothpick inserted into the center of a muffin comes out clean. Remove the muffins from the pan and transfer to a wire rack to cool. 7. Store the muffins in an airtight container at room temperature for up to 1 week or freeze for up to 3 months. Enjoy your delicious Spiced Pumpkin Muffins!

Per Serving: (1 muffin)

calories: 115 | fat: 1g | protein: 3g | carbs: 25g | fiber: 3g

Banana-Date Shake with Oats

Prep time: 15 minutes | Cook time: 0 minutes | Serves 1

1 Medjool date	2 tablespoons almond butter
10 ounces (283 g)	¼ cup rolled oats, uncooked
unsweetened vanilla almond	3 ice cubes
milk	Pinch ground cinnamon
1 small banana (fresh or	(optional)
frozen)	

1. Soak the date in hot water for 5 minutes to soften it. 2. Remove the date from the hot water, place it in a blender, and add the milk, banana, almond butter, oats, ice cubes, and cinnamon (if using). 3. Blend until smooth. 4. Enjoy your delicious and nutritious Banana-Date Shake with Oats immediately!

Per Serving:

calories: 526 | fat: 22g | protein: 19g | carbs: 72g | fiber: 11g

Strawberries and Cream Overnight Oatmeal

Prep time: 5 minutes | Cook time: 4 to 5 hours | Serves 4 to 6

Nonstick cooking spray	¼ cup maple syrup (optional)
(optional)	3 tablespoons ground
1¼ cups steel-cut oats	flaxseed
4 cups water	1 pound (454 g) fresh
1⅔ cups unsweetened plant-	strawberries, stemmed and
based milk	sliced
2 teaspoons vanilla extract	

1. Coat the inside of the slow cooker with cooking spray (if using) or line it with a slow cooker liner. 2. Place the oats, water, milk, vanilla, and maple syrup (if using) in the slow cooker. 3. Cover and cook on High for 4 to 5 hours or on Low for 8 to 9 hours. 4. When ready to serve, stir the flaxseed into the oatmeal and portion into bowls. 5. Top each serving with 3 to 5 sliced strawberries. Enjoy your delicious and convenient overnight oatmeal with a delightful strawberries and cream flavor!

Per Serving:

calories: 320 | fat: 7g | protein: 9g | carbs: 59g | fiber: 9g

Spring Breakfast Salad

Prep time: 5 minutes | Cook time: 0 minutes | Serves 2

½ cup strawberries

½ cup blueberries	juice (from 1 orange)
½ cup blackberries	1 tablespoon pure maple
½ cup raspberries	syrup (optional)
1 grapefruit, peeled and	¼ cup chopped fresh mint
segmented	¼ cup sliced almonds
3 tablespoons fresh orange	

1. In a serving bowl, combine the berries and grapefruit. 2. In a small bowl, stir together the orange juice and maple syrup (if using). Pour the syrup mixture over the fruit. Sprinkle with the mint and almonds. Serve immediately.

Per Serving:
calories: 199 | fat: 6g | protein: 4g | carbs: 34g | fiber: 8g

Overnight Oats

Prep time: 15 minutes | Cook time: 0 minutes | Serves 2

1 cup old-fashioned rolled	seeds
oats	1 cup plant-based milk
¾ cup frozen berries	1 banana, sliced
2 tablespoons raw sunflower	

1. Add the oats, berries, sunflower seeds, and milk to a storage container, glass, or mason jar. 2. Cover with a lid or aluminum foil and refrigerate overnight. 3. In the morning, mix and enjoy chilled. (No cooking or heating is necessary—the oats soften overnight.) 4. Garnish with the sliced banana to sweeten.

Per Serving:
calories: 323 | fat: 12g | protein: 15g | carbs: 58g | fiber: 11g

Cherry Pecan Granola Bars

Prep time: 10 minutes | Cook time: 45 minutes | Makes 12 bars

2 cups rolled oats	cherries
½ cup dates, pitted and	½ teaspoon ground
coarsely chopped	cinnamon
½ cup orange juice	¼ teaspoon ground allspice
¼ cup chopped pecans	Pinch salt, or to taste
1 cup fruit-sweetened dried	(optional)

1. Preheat the oven to 325ºF (165ºC). 2. Spread the oats on a 13 × 18-inch baking sheet and bake for 10 minutes, or until they start to brown. Remove from the oven and place the oats in a large mixing bowl. 3. Combine the dates and orange juice in a small saucepan and cook over medium-low heat for about 15 minutes. Pour the mixture into a blender and process until smooth and creamy. 4. Add the date mixture to the bowl with the oats and add the pecans, dried cherries, cinnamon, allspice, and salt (if using). Mix well. 5. Press the mixture into a nonstick 8 × 8-inch baking pan and bake for 20 minutes, or until the top is lightly golden. Let cool before slicing into bars.

Per Serving:
calories: 92 | fat: 2g | protein: 3g | carbs: 20g | fiber: 3g

Overnight Muesli

Prep time: 15 minutes | Cook time: 0 minutes | Serves 6

2 cups old-fashioned oats	¼ cup slivered almonds
1 cup raisins	¼ cup chopped walnuts
½ cup wheat germ	¼ cup sunflower seed
½ cup oat bran	kernels
½ cup chopped dates	7 cups almond milk or other
½ cup pepitas	dairy-free milk
¼ cup wheat bran	

1. Place all the dry ingredients in a large mixing bowl. Mix well. Pour in the milk and mix well again. 2. Cover and place in the refrigerator to sit overnight. 3. The muesli is ready to eat in the morning and keeps for 4 to 5 days.

Per Serving:
calories: 423 | fat: 17g | protein: 16g | carbs: 46g | fiber: 11g

Chocolate Cherry Oats Bowl

Prep time: 5 minutes | Cook time: 5 minutes | Serves 2

½ cup fresh or frozen	¼ cup almond flakes
cherries	2 cups water
2 tangerines	Optional Toppings:
1 cup instant oats	Crushed dark chocolate
1 scoop soy protein isolate,	Mint leaves
chocolate flavor	Cinnamon

1. In a saucepan, combine water and oats over medium heat. 2. Bring to a boil and cook the oats for about 5 minutes. 3. Turn off the heat and stir in the soy isolate until well combined. 4. Peel and section the tangerines. 5. Transfer the protein oats to a bowl, then top with almond flakes, tangerines, and cherries. 6. Serve the oats warm with optional toppings and enjoy! 7. Store any leftovers in an airtight container in the fridge for up to 2 days or freeze for up to 60 days. Thaw at room temperature before eating.

Per Serving:
calories: 349 | fat: 9g | protein: 22g | carbs: 44g | fiber: 7g

Chia Seed and Raspberry Pudding

Prep time: 5 minutes | Cook time: 0 minutes | Serves 2

1¼ cups fresh raspberries, divided	1¼ cups unsweetened vanilla almond milk
1 tablespoon maple syrup (optional)	3 tablespoons chia seeds

1. In a medium mixing bowl, mash 1 cup of raspberries with a fork; then add the maple syrup (if using) and mix well. 2. Add the almond milk and chia seeds to the bowl. Whisk together until well mixed. 3. Pour even amounts of the mixture in two glasses, cover, and let sit in the refrigerator for at least 45 minutes. 4. When ready to eat, top with the remaining ¼ cup of raspberries and enjoy cold.

Per Serving:

calories: 213 | fat: 8g | protein: 8g | carbs: 30g | fiber: 13g

Overnight Pumpkin Spice Chia Pudding

Prep time: 10 minutes | Cook time: 0 minutes | Serves 4

¾ cup chia seeds	¼ cup maple syrup (optional)
2 cups unsweetened plant-based milk	1 tablespoon pumpkin pie spice blend
1 (15-ounce / 425-g) can unsweetened pumpkin purée	1 cup water
	½ cup pecans, for serving

1. In a large bowl, whisk together the chia seeds, plant-based milk, pumpkin purée, maple syrup (if using), pumpkin pie spice, and water. 2. Divide the mixture among 4 mason jars or containers with lids. Let sit for 10 minutes. Stir each container to break up any chia clumps. Cover and refrigerate overnight to firm up. To serve, garnish each with some of the pecans.

Per Serving:

calories: 421 | fat: 23g | protein: 12g | carbs: 47g | fiber: 20g

Millet Porridge with Pumpkin and Cinnamon

Prep time: 5 minutes | Cook time: 25 minutes | Serves 2

1¼ cups unsweetened plain or vanilla almond milk	½ cup pumpkin purée
½ cup millet	Pinch ground cinnamon
½ cup golden raisins (sultanas), no sugar added	Pinch ground nutmeg (optional)

1. In a small pot, bring the almond milk to a boil. 2. Add the millet and raisins. Return to a boil; then reduce the heat to a simmer. Cover and cook for 20 minutes until the millet is tender. 3. Add the pumpkin purée and cook for 3 to 5 minutes more, just enough time to heat the porridge through. 4. Serve in small bowls and top with the cinnamon and nutmeg (if using).

Per Serving:

calories: 378 | fat: 4g | protein: 11g | carbs: 79g | fiber: 8g

Seeds, Nuts, and Fruit Baked Granola

Prep time: 10 minutes | Cook time: 40 minutes | Serves 8

7 cups old-fashioned oats (use gluten-free if desired)	1 cup coconut sugar (optional)
1 cup shredded coconut	¼ cup chia seeds
1 cup sunflower seed kernels	1 cup coconut oil (optional)
1 cup walnuts	1 cup raisins

1. Preheat the oven to 300ºF (150ºC). 2. Mix all the ingredients together except for the raisins. Spread out in a large baking pan. 3. Bake for 40 minutes. Take out of the oven every 10 minutes and stir. Return to the oven. 4. After 30 minutes, add raisins and stir. Bake for 10 more minutes. Take out of the oven and let cool. 5. Pack in airtight container. Will keep for 4 weeks.

Per Serving:

calories: 566 | fat: 32g | protein: 20g | carbs: 52g | fiber: 16g

Whole-Wheat Blueberry Muffins

Prep time: 5 minutes | Cook time: 25 minutes | Makes 8 muffins

½ cup plant-based milk	1 teaspoon vanilla extract
½ cup unsweetened applesauce	2 cups whole-wheat flour
½ cup maple syrup (optional)	½ teaspoon baking soda
	1 cup blueberries

1. Preheat the oven to 375ºF (190ºC). 2. In a large bowl, combine the milk, applesauce, and maple syrup (if desired), and vanilla. 3. Stir in the whole-wheat flour and baking soda until the batter is smooth and no dry flour remains. 4. Gently fold in the blueberries, distributing them evenly throughout the batter. 5. Fill 8 muffin cups in a muffin tin three-quarters full with the batter. 6. Bake for 25 minutes or until a knife inserted into the center of a muffin comes out clean. Allow the muffins to cool before serving. Enjoy your delicious Whole-Wheat Blueberry Muffins!

Per Serving: (1 muffin)

calories: 200 | fat: 1g | protein: 4g | carbs: 45g | fiber: 2g

Best Whole Wheat Pancakes

Prep time: 10 minutes | Cook time: 20 minutes | Serves 4

3 tablespoons ground flaxseed	1 teaspoon ground cinnamon
6 tablespoons warm water	½ teaspoon ground ginger
1½ cups whole wheat pastry flour	1½ cups unsweetened nondairy milk
½ cup rye flour	3 tablespoons pure maple syrup (optional)
2 tablespoons double-acting baking powder	1 teaspoon vanilla extract

1. In a small bowl, stir together the flaxseed and warm water. Set aside for at least 5 minutes. 2. In a large bowl, whisk together the pastry and rye flours, baking powder, cinnamon, and ginger to combine. 3. In a glass measuring cup, whisk together the milk, maple syrup (if using), and vanilla. Using a spatula, fold the wet ingredients into the dry ingredients. Fold in the soaked flaxseed until fully incorporated. 4. Heat a large skillet or nonstick griddle over medium-high heat. Working in batches, 3 to 4 pancakes at a time, add ¼-cup portions of batter to the hot skillet. Cook for 3 to 4 minutes per side, or until golden brown and no liquid batter is visible.

Per Serving: (3 pancakes)

calories: 301 | fat: 4g | protein: 10g | carbs: 57g | fiber: 10g

Peaches and Cream Overnight Oats

Prep time: 10 minutes | Cook time: 0 minutes | Serves 2

½ cup rolled oats	1 tablespoon maple syrup (optional)
1 cup light unsweetened coconut milk	Pinch of salt (optional)
½ cup peaches, fresh or frozen, diced into 1-inch pieces	2 tablespoons slivered almonds, for serving
½ teaspoon vanilla extract	2 tablespoons plain plant-based yogurt, for serving

1. In a medium bowl, combine oats, coconut milk, peaches, vanilla, maple syrup, and salt (if using). Stir well to mix all the ingredients. Cover the bowl and refrigerate overnight. 2. When ready to serve, top each serving with 1 tablespoon of slivered almonds and 1 tablespoon of plant-based yogurt. Enjoy your delicious and creamy Peaches and Cream Overnight Oats!

Per Serving:

calories: 280 | fat: 17g | protein: 7g | carbs: 27g | fiber: 4g

Hemp and Vanilla Bircher Breakfast

Prep time: 15 minutes | Cook time: 0 minutes | Serves 1

⅓ cup certified gluten-free rolled oats	(optional)
1 tablespoon hulled hemp seeds	1 cup unsweetened almond milk
1 tablespoon chia seeds	1 teaspoon pure maple syrup, or to taste (optional)
¼ teaspoon vanilla powder or pure vanilla extract	Serve:
⅛ teaspoon fine sea salt	Chopped fresh fruit
	Nut or seed butter

1. In a small sealable jar (or other container), combine the oats, hemp seeds, chia seeds, vanilla powder, sea salt, if using, and almond milk. Stir to combine. Place the lid on the container, and refrigerate for at least 4 hours but ideally overnight. 2. Retrieve and uncover the bircher breakfast after it has chilled. Add the maple syrup to the jar and give it a stir to combine. Serve with fresh fruit and a spoonful of nut or seed butter if you like.

Per Serving:

calories: 302 | fat: 12g | protein: 10g | carbs: 33g | fiber: 9g

Fruit Salad with Zesty Citrus Couscous

Prep time: 5 minutes | Cook time: 5 minutes | Serves 1

1 orange, zested and juiced	(cantaloupe or honeydew)
¼ cup whole wheat couscous or corn couscous	1 tablespoon maple syrup or coconut sugar (optional)
1 cup assorted berries (strawberries, blackberries, blueberries)	1 tablespoon fresh mint, minced (optional)
½ cup cubed or balled melon	1 tablespoon unsweetened coconut flakes

1. Put the orange juice in a small pot, add half the zest, and bring to a boil. 2. Put the dry couscous in a small bowl and pour the boiling orange juice over it. If there isn't enough juice to fully submerge the couscous, add just enough boiling water to do so. Cover the bowl with a plate or seal with wrap, and let steep for 5 minutes. 3. In a medium bowl, toss the berries and melon with the maple syrup (if using) and the rest of the zest. You can either keep the fruit cool, or heat it lightly in the small pot you used for the orange juice. 4. When the couscous is soft, remove the cover and fluff it with a fork. Top with the fruit, fresh mint, and coconut.

Per Serving:

calories: 258 | fat: 2g | protein: 4g | carbs: 59g | fiber: 7g

Chia Oat Bircher Bowl

Prep time: 10 minutes | Cook time: 0 minutes | Makes 4 cups

½ cup rolled oats

¼ cup chia seeds

¼ cup hemp seeds

2 tablespoons ground flaxseeds

½ cup whole raw almonds, soaked overnight in 2 cups filtered

water

2¾ cups filtered water

1 tablespoon vanilla extract

2 teaspoons ground cinnamon

Pinch of fine sea salt (optional)

1. Combine the oats and the chia, hemp, and flaxseeds in a medium bowl; set aside. Drain and rinse the almonds and transfer them to an upright blender. Add the 2¾ cups water, vanilla, cinnamon, and salt, if using, and blend until completely smooth, then pour into the oat mixture. Stir well to combine and set aside for 25 to 30 minutes, until thick and creamy. 2. The bowl can be eaten immediately, with any of the toppings suggested here, or stored in an airtight container in the fridge for up to 4 days. It will thicken further in the fridge.

Per Serving: (½ cup)

calories: 128 | fat: 9g | protein: 5g | carbs: 10g | fiber: 5g

Sweet Potato Pie Oatmeal

Prep time: 10 minutes | Cook time: 22 minutes | Serves 2

1 large sweet potato, peeled and diced

1 cup rolled oats

1 cup unsweetened almond milk

½ cup date molasses

½ teaspoon ground cinnamon

½ teaspoon ground ginger

¼ teaspoon orange zest

¼ teaspoon ground allspice

Pinch salt (optional)

1. Steam or boil the sweet potato until tender, approximately 10 minutes. Drain and mash the sweet potato. 2. In a small saucepan, combine the mashed sweet potato with the oats, almond milk, molasses, cinnamon, ginger, orange zest, allspice, and salt (if desired). 3. Cook the mixture over medium heat, stirring occasionally, until the oats are tender and the flavors are well combined, about 10 to 12 minutes. Serve the delicious Sweet Potato Pie Oatmeal warm and enjoy the comforting flavors of a classic pie in a wholesome breakfast!

Per Serving:

calories: 400 | fat: 3g | protein: 13g | carbs: 84g | fiber: 9g

Chapter 4 Basics

Tomato Sauce

Prep time: 10 minutes | Cook time: 40 minutes | Makes 4 cups

1 medium yellow onion, peeled and diced small	2 tablespoons minced oregano
6 cloves garlic, peeled and minced	1 (28-ounce / 794-g) can diced tomatoes, puréed
6 tablespoons minced basil	Salt, to taste (optional)

1. Place the onion in a large saucepan and sauté over medium heat for 10 minutes, adding water 1 to 2 tablespoons at a time to prevent sticking. 2. Add garlic, basil, and oregano, and cook for another 3 minutes. 3. Stir in the puréed tomatoes and salt (if using). Cover the saucepan and cook over medium-low heat for 25 minutes. Enjoy the rich and flavorful Tomato Sauce on your favorite dishes!

Per Serving: (1 cup)

calories: 48 | fat: 0g | protein: 2g | carbs: 10g | fiber: 4g

Tempeh Bacon

Prep time: 5 minutes | Cook time: 10 minutes | Serves 4

2 tablespoons soy sauce	1 (8-ounce / 227-g) package tempeh
1 tablespoon water	1 tablespoon canola oil (optional)
1 tablespoon maple syrup (optional)	
½ tablespoon liquid smoke	

1. In a medium bowl, combine soy sauce, water, maple syrup (if desired), and liquid smoke. Set aside. 2. Cut the tempeh block in half lengthwise and slice it as thinly as possible. 3. Heat oil (if desired) in a large pan over high heat. Add the tempeh in a single layer and cook for 2 minutes. Flip and cook for 2 more minutes. 4. While the tempeh is in the pan, add the liquid mixture and sauté for 3 minutes. Flip and cook for 3 more minutes or until the liquid is absorbed. 5. Serve the Tempeh Bacon immediately for the best flavor. Enjoy the smoky and savory taste!

Per Serving:

calories: 17 | fat: 11g | protein: 11g | carbs: 11g | fiber: 0g

Easy-Peasy Almond Milk

Prep time: 5 minutes | Cook time: 0 minutes | Makes 2 cups

2 to 3 tablespoons raw almond butter	stevia (or vanilla stevia), or 1 to 2 tablespoons unrefined sugar (optional)
2 cups water	¼ teaspoon pure vanilla extract (optional)
Pinch sea salt (optional)	
1 to 2 dates, or 10 drops pure	

1. Add almonds and water to a blender and blend until smooth. 2. Strain the mixture through cheesecloth or a fine-mesh sieve to remove almond fiber. 3. Store the almond milk in an airtight container in the fridge for up to 5 days. Enjoy the creamy and dairy-free goodness!

Per Serving: (1 cup)

calories: 110 | fat: 8g | protein: 3g | carbs: 5g | fiber: 2g

Chipotle Peppers in Adobo Sauce

Prep time: 30 minutes | Cook time: 20 minutes | Makes 20 to 25 peppers

1 (2 ounces / 57 g) package morita chiles (about 17 to 20)	½ teaspoon ground cumin
1 (2 ounces / 57 g) package chipotle chiles (about 10 to 12)	½ teaspoon dried oregano
	½ teaspoon dried marjoram
1 to 2 cups boiling water	¼ cup apple cider vinegar
½ onion, chopped	¼ cup rice vinegar
1 garlic clove, crushed	2 tablespoons date syrup (optional)
	2 tablespoons tomato paste

1. Roast morita and chipotle chiles in the oven, then rehydrate them in boiling water for 30 minutes. 2. Sauté onion, garlic, cumin, oregano, and marjoram in a skillet. 3. Transfer the onion mixture to a blender, add apple cider vinegar, rice vinegar, date syrup (optional), and tomato paste. 4. Blend with rehydrated chiles and their soaking liquid. 5. Cook the sauce with remaining chiles until reduced by half. Enjoy the spicy and flavorful sauce!

Per Serving:

calories: 30 | fat: 0g | protein: 1g | carbs: 6g | fiber: 2g

Tahini Dressing

Prep time: 5 minutes | Cook time: 0 minutes | Makes ½ cup

¼ cup tahini	1 teaspoon ground cumin
1 teaspoon minced garlic	1 tablespoon olive oil (optional)
3 tablespoons lemon juice	
1 tablespoon maple syrup (optional)	1 tablespoon hot water
1 teaspoon soy sauce	Pinch of salt and pepper (optional)

1. In a small bowl, whisk together all the ingredients until well combined. 2. Store the dressing in an airtight container in the fridge for up to 7 days. Enjoy this delicious and versatile dressing on salads, bowls, or as a dip!

Per Serving: (½ cup)

calories: 283 | fat: 24g | protein: 6g | carbs: 16g | fiber: 3g

Mayonnaise

Prep time: 5 minutes | Cook time: 0 minutes | Makes 1½ cups

1 (12-ounce / 340-g) package extra-firm silken tofu, drained	½ teaspoon garlic powder
	½ teaspoon salt, or to taste (optional)
1 teaspoon dry mustard	3 tablespoons red wine vinegar
½ teaspoon onion powder	

1. Combine all ingredients in the bowl of a food processor. 2. Purée until smooth and creamy. Enjoy your homemade mayo!

Per Serving: (½ cup)

calories: 110 | fat: 6g | protein: 11g | carbs: 3g | fiber: 0g

Herbed Millet Pizza Crust

Prep time: 5 minutes | Cook time: 40 minutes | Makes 1 large thin-crust pizza crust

½ cup coarsely ground millet	¼ teaspoon sea salt (optional)
1½ cups water	
1 tablespoon mixed dried Italian herbs	1 to 2 tablespoons nutritional yeast

1. Preheat your oven to 350ºF (180ºC) and line an 8-inch-round pie dish or springform pan with parchment paper for easy removal after cooking. Ensure the pan is nonstick or use parchment paper to prevent sticking. 2. In a small pot, combine the millet, water, and a pinch of salt. Bring it to a boil, then cover and simmer for 15 to 20 minutes, stirring occasionally to prevent sticking. For enhanced flavor, you can cook the millet with dried herbs or add them in after cooking. 3. Once the millet is cooked, add the optional salt (if desired) and nutritional yeast for added flavor. Spread the seasoned millet evenly in the prepared pan, covering the entire surface. 4. Bake the crust in the preheated oven for about 20 minutes or until the edges become lightly browned. Once cooked, allow the crust to cool slightly before using it as a base for your favorite pizza toppings. Enjoy this wholesome and nutritious gluten-free alternative!

Per Serving: (1 crust)

calories: 378 | fat: 4g | protein: 11g | carbs: 72g | fiber: 8g

Tofu Sour Cream

Prep time: 5 minutes | Cook time: 0 minutes | Makes 1½ cups

1 (12-ounce / 340-g) package extra-firm silken tofu, drained	juice
	1 tablespoon red wine vinegar
1 tablespoon fresh lemon	Salt, to taste (optional)

1. Combine all ingredients in a blender and purée until smooth and creamy. 2. Chill until ready to serve. Enjoy the dairy-free alternative!

Per Serving: (½ cup)

calories: 105 | fat: 6g | protein: 11g | carbs: 2g | fiber: 0g

5-Minute Tofu Cheese Sauce

Prep time: 5 minutes | Cook time: 0 minutes | Makes about 2 cups

1 (12-ounce / 340-g) package silken tofu	2 teaspoons Dijon mustard
½ cup nutritional yeast	1 tablespoon white wine vinegar
1½ teaspoons onion powder	1 teaspoon salt (optional)
½ teaspoon garlic powder	½ cup unsweetened plant-based milk
¼ teaspoon paprika	

1. Place the tofu, nutritional yeast, onion powder, garlic powder, paprika, mustard, vinegar, salt (if using), and milk into a blender or food processor. Blend for 30 to 60 seconds until the mixture is well combined and creamy. 2. Heat the sauce on the stove or in the microwave until warmed to your desired temperature. This versatile and flavorful sauce is perfect for drizzling over pasta, vegetables, or as a dip for your favorite snacks. Store any leftovers in the refrigerator for up to 4 days. Enjoy the creamy goodness!

Per Serving:

calories: 54 | fat: 2g | protein: 7g | carbs: 4g | fiber: 2g

Croutons

Prep time: 5 minutes | Cook time: 15 minutes | Serves 4

½ day-old baguette, sliced	½ tablespoon garlic salt
2 tablespoons olive oil	(optional)
(optional)	

1. Preheat the oven to 350ºF (180ºC). 2. Brush the baguette slices with the olive oil and sprinkle with the garlic salt, if desired. 3. Cut the bread into cubes, place on a baking sheet, and bake for 10 to 15 minutes or until golden brown. 4. Allow the croutons to cool before serving. 5. The croutons are best if served immediately after baking.

Per Serving:

calories: 94 | fat: 7g | protein: 1g | carbs: 7g | fiber: 0g

Fresh Tomato Salsa

Prep time: 15 minutes | Cook time: 0 minutes | Makes about 4 cups

3 large ripe tomatoes, diced small	remove the seeds)
	2 cloves garlic, peeled and minced
1 small red onion, peeled and diced small	3 tablespoons fresh lime juice
½ cup chopped cilantro	Salt, to taste (optional)
1 to 2 jalapeño peppers, minced (for less heat,	

1. Combine all ingredients in a large bowl and mix well. Store refrigerated until ready to serve.

Per Serving: (1 cup)

calories: 38 | fat: 0g | protein: 1g | carbs: 8g | fiber: 2g

Piecrust

Prep time: 10 minutes | Cook time: 0 minutes | Serves 4

1 cup all-purpose flour, plus more for rolling	for later (optional)
	½ teaspoon lemon juice
½ teaspoon baking powder	3½ tablespoons plant-based milk
¼ teaspoon salt (optional)	
2 tablespoons canola oil, plus more if storing dough	4 tablespoons water

1. In a medium bowl, thoroughly mix all the ingredients using a wooden spoon until a ball of dough forms. 2. Wrap the dough in plastic wrap and refrigerate for 1 hour. 3. If using immediately, dust a work surface with flour, place the chilled dough down, and roll it out into a thin, flat 11-inch circle using a lightly floured rolling pin. Transfer the rolled dough to a 9-inch pie dish. Fill with your choice of fillings and bake according to the recipe's instructions. 4. If not using immediately, cover the dough's exterior with 1 teaspoon of oil (if desired) to prevent drying out. Place the lightly oiled dough in a medium bowl, tightly cover it with plastic wrap or place it in an airtight container, and refrigerate for up to 7 days. Enjoy your homemade piecrust in a delicious pie of your choice!

Per Serving:

calories: 183 | fat: 8g | protein: 4g | carbs: 25g | fiber: 1g

Chili Powder

Prep time: 15 minutes | Cook time: 0 minutes | Makes about ½ cup

3 arbol chiles	(not ground)
5 guajillo chiles	2 tablespoons garlic powder
5 California chiles	1 tablespoon dried oregano
2 tablespoons cumin seeds	1 tablespoon onion powder

1. Heat a cast-iron skillet over high heat. As the skillet heats up, remove and discard the stems and seeds from the arbol, guajillo, and California chiles. 2. Place the chiles in the hot, dry skillet and roast for 3 to 5 minutes, turning occasionally, until the color slightly changes and the chiles become softer. Transfer the chiles to a blender or food processor. 3. Put the cumin seeds in the hot skillet and toast until they begin popping. Immediately transfer them to the blender, along with the garlic powder, oregano, and onion powder. 4. Cover tightly and blend into a fine powder. Allow the powder to settle for 2 to 3 minutes before removing the lid. Store in a cool, dry location for up to 6 months.

Per Serving:

calories: 7 | fat: 0g | protein: 0g | carbs: 1g | fiber: 0g

Lemon-Tahini Dressing

Prep time: 5 minutes | Cook time: 0 minutes | Serves 8

¼ cup fresh lemon juice	½ cup gluten-free tahini
1 teaspoon maple syrup	¼ teaspoon salt (optional)
(optional)	⅛ teaspoon black pepper
1 small garlic clove, chopped	¼ to ½ cup water

1. Pulse the lemon juice, sugar, garlic, tahini, salt (if desired), and pepper in a high-speed blender to combine. Slowly add the water, starting with ¼ cup, until it reaches the desired consistency. Refrigerate in an airtight container for up to 5 days.

Per Serving:

calories: 94 | fat: 8g | protein: 3g | carbs: 4g | fiber: 1g

Spicy Cilantro Pesto

Prep time: 10 minutes | Cook time: 0 minutes | Makes about 1 cup

2 cups packed cilantro	Zest and juice of 1 lime
¼ cup hulled sunflower seeds, toasted (optional)	Salt, to taste (optional)
1 jalapeño pepper, coarsely chopped (for less heat, remove the seeds)	½ package extra-firm silken tofu (about 6 ounces / 170 g), drained
4 cloves garlic, peeled and chopped	¼ cup nutritional yeast (optional)

1. In a food processor, combine cilantro, sunflower seeds (optional), jalapeño pepper, garlic, lime zest, lime juice, salt (optional), tofu, and nutritional yeast (optional). 2. Purée the mixture until smooth and creamy. 3. Enjoy the flavorful and spicy cilantro pesto!

Per Serving: (¼ cup)

calories: 143 | fat: 8g | protein: 11g | carbs: 10g | fiber: 5g

Pure Nut Mylk

Prep time: 2 minutes | Cook time: 0 minutes | Makes 3 cups

1 cup raw, unsalted nuts (almonds, hazelnuts, Brazil nuts, pecans, macadamias, walnuts)	3 cups purified water for blending, plus more if desired

1. Soak the nuts overnight in 2 to 3 cups of water. 2. Drain and rinse the nuts, then blend them with 3 cups of purified water until smooth. 3. Strain the mixture through cheesecloth or a nut milk bag, squeezing out as much liquid as possible. 4. Adjust the consistency by adding more purified water if desired. 5. Store the nut mylk in a glass jar in the refrigerator for 3 to 4 days. Enjoy the creamy and nutritious Pure Nut Mylk in your favorite recipes!

Per Serving:

calories: 276 | fat: 23g | protein: 10g | carbs: 10g | fiber: 6g

Lime-Cumin Dressing

Prep time: 5 minutes | Cook time: 0 minutes | Serves 4

1 teaspoon ground cumin	juice
1 teaspoon coconut sugar (optional)	1 tablespoon apple cider vinegar
¼ teaspoon salt (optional)	2 teaspoons extra virgin olive oil (optional)
3 tablespoons fresh lime	

1. In a medium jar with a tight-fitting lid, combine the cumin, sugar, and salt (if desired). Whisk in the fresh lime juice and vinegar until well combined. 2. Optionally, you can slowly add the oil in a steady stream while whisking to emulsify the dressing. Refrigerate the dressing for up to 4 days. Remember to shake the jar to combine the flavors before each use. This zesty and flavorful dressing is a delightful addition to salads, roasted vegetables, and more. Enjoy the tangy goodness!

Per Serving:

calories: 28 | fat: 2g | protein: 0g | carbs: 2g | fiber: 2g

Plant-Based Fish Sauce

Prep time: 10 minutes | Cook time: 20 minutes | Makes 3 to 4 cups

4 cups water	¼ cup low-sodium soy sauce, tamari, or coconut aminos
1 (4-by-8-inch) sheet of kombu	
½ cup dried shiitake mushrooms	3 garlic cloves, crushed
	2 teaspoons rice vinegar

1. In a medium saucepan, combine water, kombu, mushrooms, soy sauce, garlic, and vinegar. Bring the mixture to a boil, then reduce the heat to low. 2. Cover and simmer for 15 to 20 minutes. Remove from the heat. Allow the mixture to steep overnight or for at least 8 hours, keeping it covered. 3. Strain the liquid to remove any solids and discard them. Store the plant-based fish sauce in a glass bottle in the refrigerator for up to 3 weeks. Shake well before each use. Enjoy this flavorful and vegan-friendly alternative in your favorite recipes!

Per Serving:

calories: 4 | fat: 0g | protein: 0g | carbs: 1g | fiber: 0g

Mama Mia Marinara Sauce

Prep time: 10 minutes | Cook time: 2 to 3 hours | Makes about 7 cups

1 medium onion, diced	2 tablespoons Italian seasoning, or 1 tablespoon each dried basil and dried oregano
5 garlic cloves, minced	
2 (28-ounce / 794-g) cans no-salt-added crushed tomatoes	
	Ground black pepper
½ cup red wine	Salt (optional)

1. Put the onion, garlic, and tomatoes in the slow cooker. Swirl the wine in the empty tomato cans and pour everything into the slow cooker. Add the Italian seasoning, pepper, and salt (if using). Stir to combine. 2. Cover and cook on High for 2 to 3 hours or on Low for 4 to 5 hours.

Per Serving:

calories: 30 | fat: 0g | protein: 1g | carbs: 4g | fiber: 1g

Buckwheat Sesame Milk

Prep time: 5 minutes | Cook time: 0 minutes | Makes 4 cups

1 cup cooked buckwheat
1 tablespoon tahini, or other nut or seed butter
1 teaspoon pure vanilla extract (optional)
2 to 3 dates, or 15 drops pure stevia (or vanilla stevia), or 2 to 3 tablespoons unrefined sugar (optional)
3 cups water

1. Combine all ingredients in a blender and blend until smooth. 2. Strain the mixture through cheesecloth or a fine-mesh sieve to remove any fiber. 3. Store the milk in an airtight container in the fridge for up to 5 days. Enjoy the nutty flavor and plant-based goodness!

Per Serving: (1 cup)

calories: 76 | fat: 2g | protein: 2g | carbs: 12g | fiber: 1g

Apple Cider Vinaigrette

Prep time: 5 minutes | Cook time: 0 minutes | Makes ½ cup

2 tablespoons apple cider vinegar	(optional)
¼ cup olive oil (optional)	1 teaspoon minced garlic
½ tablespoon Dijon mustard	Pinch of salt (optional)
1 tablespoon maple syrup	Freshly ground pepper, to taste

1. Whisk together all the ingredients in a small bowl until well combined. 2. Transfer the vinaigrette to an airtight container and store it in the fridge for up to 7 days. Enjoy the tangy and flavorful dressing on your favorite salads!

Per Serving: (½ cup)

calories: 272 | fat: 27g | protein: 0g | carbs: 8g | fiber: 0g

Maple-Dijon Dressing

Prep time: 5 minutes | Cook time: 0 minutes | Serves 4

¼ cup apple cider vinegar	¼ teaspoon black pepper
2 tablespoons maple syrup	2 tablespoons water
2 teaspoons gluten-free Dijon mustard	Salt (optional)

1. Combine the vinegar, maple syrup (if desired), mustard, pepper, and water in a small jar with a tight-fitting lid. 2. Season with salt to taste, if desired. 3. Refrigerate the dressing for up to 5 days. This delightful dressing adds a perfect balance of sweetness and tanginess to your salads or drizzled over roasted vegetables. Enjoy!

Per Serving:

calories: 31 | fat: 0g | protein: 0g | carbs: 7g | fiber: 0g

Quinoa

Prep time: 5 minutes | Cook time: 5 minutes | Makes 3 cups

1 cup quinoa	1½ cups vegetable broth

1. Rinse the quinoa in cold water using a fine-mesh strainer. 2. Put the quinoa and broth into the pressure cooker and cook on high pressure for 5 minutes. 3. Let the pressure out, remove the lid, and fluff the quinoa with a fork. 4. Store in an airtight container in the fridge for up to 5 days.

Per Serving: (1 cup)

calories: 214 | fat: 3g | protein: 8g | carbs: 38g | fiber: 4g

Plant-Based Parmesan

Prep time: 5 minutes | Cook time: 0 minutes | Makes 1 heaping cup

1 cup raw cashews	¾ teaspoon garlic powder
⅓ cup nutritional yeast	½ teaspoon salt (optional)

1. In a blender or food processor, combine cashews, nutritional yeast, garlic powder, and salt (if using). 2. Blend on medium-high until the mixture reaches a texture similar to grated parmesan cheese. You may need to stop and start the blender or food processor a few times to ensure even blending. 3. Transfer the plant-based parmesan to a glass or plastic container and store it in the refrigerator for up to 1 month. Enjoy this delicious and dairy-free alternative sprinkled on your favorite dishes!

Per Serving:

calories: 219 | fat: 15g | protein: 11g | carbs: 14g | fiber: 4g

Mango-Orange Dressing

Prep time: 5 minutes | Cook time: 0 minutes | Serves 8

1 cup diced mango	1 teaspoon coconut sugar (optional)
½ cup orange juice	¼ teaspoon salt (optional)
2 tablespoons fresh lime juice	2 tablespoons chopped cilantro
2 tablespoons gluten-free rice vinegar	

1. Process the mango, orange juice, lime juice, rice vinegar, sugar, and salt (if desired) in a blender until smooth. Stir in the cilantro. Refrigerate in an airtight container for up to 2 days.

Per Serving:

calories: 23 | fat: 0g | protein: 0g | carbs: 6g | fiber: 0g

Green Split Peas

Prep time: 5 minutes | Cook time: 45 minutes | Makes 2 cups

1 cup split peas, rinsed	1½ cups water

1. Put the split peas and water into a large pot with a lid. 2. Over high heat, bring to a boil. 3. Cover the pot with the lid and reduce the heat to low. 4. Simmer for 45 minutes. 5. Store in an airtight container in the fridge for up to 5 days.

Per Serving: (1 cup)

calories: 347 | fat: 1g | protein: 24g | carbs: 63g | fiber: 25g

Green on Greens Dressing

Prep time: 10 minutes | Cook time: 0 minutes | Serves 10

¾ cup water, plus extra as needed	1 tablespoon apple cider vinegar
½ cup chopped flat-leaf parsley	2 umeboshi plums, pitted and roughly chopped
¼ cup tahini	1 teaspoon reduced-sodium tamari
1 scallion, sliced	

1. Process all the ingredients in a blender until smooth. The dressing will thicken upon sitting, so add additional water as desired before serving. Refrigerate in an airtight container for up to 2 days.

Per Serving:

calories: 44 | fat: 3g | protein: 2g | carbs: 3g | fiber: 1g

20-Minute Cashew Cheese Sauce

Prep time: 5 minutes | Cook time: 15 minutes | Makes about 3 cups

½ cup raw cashews	yeast
1 cup peeled and diced potatoes	1 tablespoon lemon juice
¼ cup diced carrots	1 teaspoon miso paste
¼ cup diced onions	½ teaspoon garlic powder
3 cups water	½ teaspoon dry mustard
4 tablespoons nutritional	Pinch paprika
	Ground black pepper
	Salt (optional)

1. Soak the cashews for 30 to 60 minutes in very hot (boiled) water before use in order for your sauce to be creamy and delicious. You can omit this step if you have a high-speed blender. 2. In a medium pot, combine the potatoes, carrots, and onion and cover with the water. Bring to a boil and cook for about 15 minutes, until the vegetables are tender and easily mushed with a fork. 3. While the vegetables are boiling, drain the cashews if you soaked them. Transfer them to a blender or food processor and add the nutritional yeast, lemon juice, miso paste, garlic powder, mustard, and paprika. Season with pepper and salt (if using). 4. When the vegetables are cooked, reserve 1 cup of cooking water and add it to the blender along with the cooked vegetables. Blend for 30 to 60 seconds, until smooth. This will keep for up to 4 days in the refrigerator.

Per Serving:

calories: 55 | fat: 3g | protein: 3g | carbs: 6g | fiber: 1g

Quinoa Mylk

Prep time: 5 minutes | Cook time: 20 minutes | Makes 4 cups

½ cup uncooked quinoa	blending
4 cups purified water, for	4 dates

1. Soak the quinoa overnight in 1 cup of water. Before cooking, drain through a fine strainer and rinse until the water runs clear. 2. To cook, in a medium saucepan, bring another 2 cups of water to a boil. Add the quinoa and bring to a second boil, then cover and simmer over low heat for 15 minutes. Remove from the heat and allow the quinoa to cool. Place the cooled quinoa in a blender with the 4 cups of purified water. Blend on high speed for 1 to 3 minutes, or until smooth. 3. Strain the blended quinoa mixture, using a cheesecloth or a nut milk bag. The milk will strain through slowly on its own, but you can gently squeeze and massage the bottom of the cloth to speed up the process. 4. Pour the quinoa mylk back in the blender, add the dates and blend until smooth. 5. Transfer the quinoa mylk to a glass jar with a tight lid and store in the fridge for 3 to 4 days.

Per Serving:

calories: 98 | fat: 1g | protein: 3g | carbs: 19g | fiber: 2g

Cauliflower Béchamel

Prep time: 15 minutes | Cook time: 30 minutes | Makes about 3½ cups

1 large head cauliflower, cut into florets (about 3 cups)	2 teaspoons minced thyme
Unsweetened plain almond milk, as needed	¼ cup finely chopped basil
1 medium yellow onion, peeled and diced small	¼ cup nutritional yeast (optional)
2 cloves garlic, peeled and minced	¼ teaspoon ground nutmeg
	Salt and freshly ground black pepper, to taste

1. Boil cauliflower until tender, then purée it with almond milk if needed for creaminess. 2. Sauté onion, garlic, thyme, and basil in a skillet. Add nutritional yeast, nutmeg, salt, and pepper. 3. Blend the onion mixture with the cauliflower purée until smooth, adding water for desired consistency if necessary. Enjoy your creamy and flavorful Cauliflower Béchamel!

Per Serving: (½ cup)

calories: 38 | fat: 0g | protein: 3g | carbs: 6g | fiber: 3g

Chapter 5 Beans and Grains

Sweet Potato Tacos

Prep time: 15 minutes | Cook time: 15 minutes | Makes 6 tacos

2 cups cooked or canned black beans	seasoning
1 (7-ounce / 198-g) pack textured soy mince	1 cup water
3 small cubed sweet potatoes	Optional Toppings:
6 whole wheat taco shells	Red onion
¼ cup Mexican chorizo	Lemon slices
	Jalapeño slices

1. If using dry beans, soak and cook 1½ cups of dry black beans. 2. Cook the sweet potato cubes in a pot of water over medium-high heat for about 15 minutes until soft. Drain and set aside. 3. In a nonstick frying pan, cook the soy mince, black beans, chorizo seasoning, and water. Stir continuously until cooked. 4. Add the cooked sweet potato cubes and stir. 5. Remove from heat and let it sit for 5 minutes. 6. Fill 6 taco shells with the sweet potato mixture, and serve with optional toppings. 7. Store the sweet potato mixture in an airtight container in the fridge for up to 3 days or freeze for up to 30 days. Reheat using a microwave, toaster oven, or nonstick frying pan.

Per Serving:

calories: 202 | fat: 3g | protein: 13g | carbs: 29g | fiber: 9g

Baked Falafel

Prep time: 15 minutes | Cook time: 30 minutes | Serves 6

1 cup dried chickpeas	1½ tablespoons chickpea flour or wheat flour (if gluten is not a concern)
½ cup packed chopped fresh parsley	
½ cup packed chopped fresh cilantro (or parsley if preferred)	2 teaspoons ground cumin
	1 teaspoon ground coriander
	½ teaspoon baking powder
½ cup chopped yellow onion	2 tablespoons freshly squeezed lemon juice
3 garlic cloves, peeled	

1. In a large bowl, soak the dried chickpeas in water overnight. Drain. 2. Preheat the oven to 375°F (190°C) and line a baking sheet with parchment paper. 3. In a blender or food processor, combine the soaked chickpeas, parsley, cilantro, onion, garlic, flour, cumin, coriander, baking powder, and lemon juice. Pulse until well combined but not smooth. 4. Using a cookie scoop or spoons, form the falafel mixture into 20 balls and place them on the baking sheet. Flatten each ball slightly. 5. Bake for 15 minutes, then flip and bake for another 10 to 15 minutes until lightly browned. 6. Store in an airtight container in the refrigerator for up to 1 week or freeze for up to 1 month.

Per Serving:

calories: 129 | fat: 2g | protein: 7g | carbs: 22g | fiber: 6g

Cuban-Style Black Beans with Cilantro Rice

Prep time: 20 minutes | Cook time: 1 hour 30 minutes | Serves 4

Black Beans:	stems
1 pound (454 g) black beans, soaked overnight	2 tablespoons apple cider vinegar
2 tablespoons ground cumin	½ teaspoon freshly ground white or black pepper
1 large onion, peeled and diced	3 tablespoons chopped cilantro leaves
2 bay leaves	1 medium tomato, chopped (about 1 cup)
3 cloves garlic, peeled and minced	
3 celery stalks, diced	Salt, to taste (optional)
3 medium carrots, peeled and diced	Cilantro Rice:
	1 cup brown rice
1 red bell pepper, seeded and diced	1 tablespoon low-sodium light brown miso paste
2 tablespoons minced oregano	2 tablespoons finely chopped cilantro leaves
1 cup finely chopped cilantro	

1. In a large pot, combine the beans, cumin, onion, bay leaves, garlic, celery, carrots, red pepper, oregano, cilantro stems, and water. Bring to a boil, then simmer for 90 minutes until the beans are tender. Remove and mash a quarter of the beans, then return them to the pot. Stir in apple cider vinegar, pepper, cilantro leaves, and tomato. Season with salt if desired and remove bay leaves. 2. For the cilantro rice, combine rice, water, and miso paste in a saucepan. Bring to a boil, then simmer covered for 20 minutes. Continue to simmer for another 30 minutes, then fluff the rice and stir in cilantro. 3. Serve the cilantro rice on individual plates and top with the prepared black beans. Enjoy!

Per Serving:

calories: 432 | fat: 3g | protein: 18g | carbs: 85g | fiber: 13g

Spicy Chickpeas and Fennel

Prep time: 15 minutes | Cook time: 35 minutes | Serves 4

1 large yellow onion, peeled and chopped	1 teaspoon crushed red pepper flakes
1 large fennel bulb, trimmed and thinly sliced	1 (28-ounce / 794-g) can diced tomatoes
4 cloves garlic, peeled and minced	4 cups cooked chickpeas, or 2 (15-ounce / 425-g) cans, drained and rinsed
1 tablespoon minced oregano	Chopped flat-leaf Italian parsley
1½ teaspoons ground fennel seeds	

1. Sauté onion and fennel in a large saucepan over medium heat until tender. Add water as needed to prevent sticking. 2. Stir in garlic, oregano, fennel seeds, and crushed red pepper flakes and cook for 3 minutes. Add tomatoes and chickpeas, bring to a boil, then reduce heat and simmer covered for 20 minutes. Serve garnished with parsley. Enjoy!

Per Serving:

calories: 343 | fat: 5g | protein: 17g | carbs: 61g | fiber: 19g

Miso Millet "Polenta" with Green Onions

Prep time: 10 minutes | Cook time: 15 minutes | Serves 4

⅓ cup plus 2 teaspoons coconut oil, divided (optional)	(optional)
	1 cup millet
½ cup green onions, white and green parts, chopped, plus extra for garnish	2 leeks, white and light-green parts only, chopped
	3 cups vegetable stock
Generous pinch of salt	2 teaspoons mellow or light miso

1. Heat coconut oil in a medium saucepan over medium heat. Add chopped green onions and fry until bright green and fragrant, about 15 to 20 seconds. Transfer the oil and green onions to a blender and blend until creamy. Set aside. 2. Grind millet in a food processor or blender until coarse flour-like texture. Set aside. 3. In the same saucepan, heat oil and cook leeks until tender. Add vegetable stock and miso, and bring to a boil. Gradually whisk in ground millet flour until thick and cooked like polenta. 4. Serve the millet polenta hot, drizzled with green onion oil and topped with chopped green onions. Enjoy!

Per Serving:

calories: 388 | fat: 20g | protein: 7g | carbs: 46g | fiber: 5g

Chickpea Pâté

Prep time: 10 minutes | Cook time: 0 minutes | Serves 4

1 cup whole raw nuts, toasted	½ cup filtered water
2 tablespoons extra-virgin olive oil, plus more for drizzling (optional)	1 teaspoon fine sea salt, plus more to taste (optional)
	½ teaspoon grated or pressed garlic
1 (15½-ounce / 439-g) can chickpeas, drained and rinsed well	½ teaspoon raw apple cider vinegar

1. In a food processor, combine nuts and oil, blending until smooth and runny, scraping down the sides as needed. This may take a few minutes. 2. Add chickpeas, water, salt (if using), garlic, and vinegar to the food processor. Blend until completely smooth, adjusting the consistency with more cooking liquid or water if needed. 3. Taste and add more salt if desired. Serve the pâté drizzled with olive oil, or store it in an airtight container in the fridge for up to 4 days. Enjoy your delicious Chickpea Pâté!

Per Serving:

calories: 321 | fat: 22g | protein: 11g | carbs: 23g | fiber: 7g

Mac 'N' Mince

Prep time: 15 minutes | Cook time: 10 minutes | Serves 4

2 cups whole wheat macaroni	pepper seasoning
	½ cup water
1 (7-ounce / 198-g) pack textured soy mince	2 tablespoons turmeric (optional)
½ cup tahini	Optional Toppings:
¼ cup nutritional yeast	Sun-dried tomatoes
2 tablespoons lemon garlic	Crispy onions

1. Cook the macaroni and set it aside. 2. In a nonstick deep frying pan, cook the soy mince with ¼ cup of water over medium-high heat. 3. Stir fry the soy mince until cooked and most of the water evaporates. 4. Add tahini, ¼ cup of water, nutritional yeast, lemon garlic pepper seasoning, and optional turmeric to the soy mince. 5. Cook a little longer, stirring continuously until well combined. 6. Mix in the cooked macaroni with the soy mince. 7. Divide between two plates, serve with optional toppings, and enjoy! 8. Store in an airtight container in the fridge for up to 3 days or in the freezer for up to 30 days. Reheat using a microwave, toaster oven, or frying pan.

Per Serving:

calories: 454 | fat: 20g | protein: 25g | carbs: 42g | fiber: 10g

Smoked Tofu and Beans Bowl

Prep time: 10 minutes | Cook time: 15 minutes | Serves 2

1 cup cooked or canned black beans	sweet corn
1 (7-ounce / 198-g) pack smoked tofu, cubed	¼ cup lemon juice
1 small Hass avocado, peeled and stoned	Optional Toppings: Jalapeño slices
2 cups cooked or canned	Fresh cilantro
	Red onion

1. Soak and cook ⅓ cup of dry black beans if using. 2. Preheat the oven to 350ºF (180ºC) and line a baking sheet with parchment paper. 3. Bake the tofu cubes on the baking sheet for 10 minutes or until slightly browned and dry. 4. Let the tofu cubes cool for 5 minutes. 5. Cut half of the peeled avocado into cubes and the other half into slices. 6. In a large salad bowl, combine the tofu cubes, black beans, avocado cubes, and corn. Stir well until evenly mixed. 7. If needed, divide between two bowls. Drizzle 2 tablespoons of lemon juice on each bowl and garnish with avocado slices. Serve with optional toppings. 8. Store the tofu and beans in an airtight container in the fridge for up to 2 days or freeze for up to 60 days. Enjoy your Smoked Tofu and Beans Bowl!

Per Serving:

calories: 401 | fat: 6g | protein: 21g | carbs: 64g | fiber: 20g

Roasted Beet Biryani

Prep time: 15 minutes | Cook time: 40 minutes | Serves 4

6 cups water, plus 5 tablespoons and more as needed	1 tablespoon grated peeled fresh ginger
2 cups basmati rice, rinsed well	1 large beet, peeled and finely chopped
1 teaspoon ground cardamom	3 carrots, diced
½ teaspoon cayenne pepper	1 tablespoon yellow (mellow) miso paste
¼ teaspoon ground cinnamon	Oil, for coating (optional)
¼ teaspoon ground aniseed	1 cup green peas
¼ teaspoon ground turmeric	1 (15-ounce /425-g) can chickpeas, drained and rinsed
1 yellow onion, diced	
3 garlic cloves, minced	¼ cup packed chopped fresh cilantro, plus more for garnish
1 (4-ounce / 113-g) can diced green chiles	

1. Preheat the oven to 400ºF (205ºC). 2. Parcook the rice by boiling 6 cups of water in a large pot, then adding the rice and cooking for 10 minutes. Strain the rice using a fine-mesh sieve, lightly rinse, and set aside. 3. In a small bowl, mix cardamom, cayenne pepper, cinnamon, aniseed, and turmeric with 2 tablespoons of water. Set aside. 4. Sauté onion, garlic, and 1 tablespoon of water in a pot over medium heat for 5 minutes until well browned. Add water as needed to prevent burning. 5. Stir in the soaked spices and cook for 1 minute. Add green chiles and ginger, cook for 30 seconds more. 6. Add beet, carrots, and 2 tablespoons of water. Sauté for 3 minutes, then stir in miso paste and turn off the heat. 7. Lightly coat a 9-by-13-inch baking dish with oil if using. Layer half the rice in the dish, then top with the beet and carrot mixture, peas, and chickpeas. Sprinkle cilantro evenly on top. Add the remaining rice and cover with foil. 8. Bake for 15 minutes, then lightly mix, garnish with cilantro, and serve. Enjoy your Roasted Beet Biryani!

Per Serving:

calories: 547 | fat: 3g | protein: 18g | carbs: 112g | fiber: 9g

Oil-Free Rice-and-Vegetable Stir-Fry

Prep time: 5 minutes | Cook time: 15 minutes | Serves 4

2 cups fresh or frozen green peas	water
2 cups fresh or frozen green beans	1 teaspoon garlic powder
¼ cup vegetable broth or	1 teaspoon onion powder
	4 cups cooked brown rice

1. Heat a medium saucepan over medium heat. 2. Add peas, green beans, broth, garlic powder, and onion powder. Cover and cook for 8 minutes until crisp-tender, stirring occasionally and adding more broth/water if needed to prevent sticking. 3. Uncover and stir in cooked brown rice. Cook for 5 more minutes, stirring occasionally. Serve and enjoy!

Per Serving:

calories: 233 | fat: 2g | protein: 8g | carbs: 48g | fiber: 7g

Basic Polenta

Prep time: 2 minutes | Cook time: 30 minutes | Serves 4 to 6

1½ cups coarse cornmeal	(optional)
¾ teaspoon salt, or to taste	

1. Boil 5 cups of water in a large saucepan. Gradually whisk in the cornmeal. 2. Stir the mixture constantly and cook until it becomes thick and creamy, approximately 30 minutes. 3. Add salt to taste if desired. Serve immediately or pour the polenta into a pan and refrigerate until set, which takes about 1 hour. Enjoy!

Per Serving:

calories: 145 | fat: 0g | protein: 2g | carbs: 31g | fiber: 1g

Farro Tabbouleh

Prep time: 15 minutes | Cook time: 30 minutes | Serves 6

2½ cups water or vegetable broth

1 cup farro, soaked overnight and drained

3 scallions, sliced thin

1 English cucumber, diced

1 red or yellow bell pepper, finely diced

1 bunch flat-leaf parsley

leaves, chopped

Handful mint leaves, chopped

Grated zest and juice of 2 lemons

¼ cup vegetable broth

¼ teaspoon salt (optional)

⅛ teaspoon black pepper

1. In a medium saucepan, combine water and farro. Bring it to a boil, then reduce the heat to low, cover, and cook until the farro is al dente, approximately 25 minutes. 2. Let the farro cool for 10 minutes, then transfer it to a large bowl. Add the remaining ingredients and toss to combine. Serve immediately, or refrigerate for up to 2 days (note that the herbs may discolor). Enjoy your delicious Farro Tabbouleh!

Per Serving:

calories: 115 | fat: 1g | protein: 4g | carbs: 26g | fiber: 5g

Fancy Rice

Prep time: 10 minutes | Cook time: 40 minutes | Serves 4

1 cup uncooked wild and brown rice blend, rinsed

2 teaspoons virgin olive oil (optional)

1 teaspoon apple cider vinegar

½ teaspoon ground coriander

¼ teaspoon ground sumac

¼ cup unsweetened dried

cranberries

¼ cup chopped fresh flat-leaf parsley

2 green onions, thinly sliced

Salt and pepper, to taste (optional)

¼ cup almonds, chopped, for garnish

1. In a medium saucepan, place the wild and brown rice blend and cover it with cold water by 1 inch. Bring to a boil, then reduce the heat to a simmer, and cover. Cook the rice for 40 minutes or until all the liquid is absorbed. Let the rice sit for 5 minutes, then fluff it with a fork and transfer it to a medium bowl. 2. Add olive oil, apple cider vinegar, coriander, sumac, dried cranberries, parsley, green onions, and optional salt and pepper to the rice. Gently toss to combine. Garnish the rice with chopped almonds and serve warm. Enjoy your Fancy Rice!

Per Serving:

calories: 252 | fat: 7g | protein: 5g | carbs: 25g | fiber: 3g

Red Lentil Dahl

Prep time: 15 minutes | Cook time: 15 minutes | Serves 2

2 cups cooked or canned red lentils

1 cup canned or fresh tomato cubes

2 tablespoons curry spices

¼ cup shredded coconut

¼ cup water

Optional Toppings:

Lime juice

Cherry tomatoes

Nigella seeds

1. If using dry lentils, soak and cook ⅔ cup of lentils if needed. 2. In a large pot over medium heat, add tomato cubes, shredded coconut, and water. 3. Cook for a few minutes until everything is cooked, then add curry spices and stir thoroughly. 4. Add the lentils and mix well. 5. Cook for a couple more minutes, then lower the heat to a simmer. 6. Let the dahl simmer for about 15 minutes, stirring occasionally. 7. Turn off the heat, let it cool down for a minute. 8. Divide the dahl between 2 bowls, garnish with optional toppings, and serve. Enjoy your Red Lentil Dahl! 9. Store any leftovers in an airtight container in the fridge for up to 2 days or in the freezer for up to 30 days. Reheat in the microwave or a saucepan as needed.

Per Serving:

calories: 330 | fat: 7g | protein: 19g | carbs: 46g | fiber: 18g

Nut-Crusted Tofu

Prep time: 10 minutes | Cook time: 20 minutes | Makes 8 slices

½ cup roasted, shelled pistachios

¼ cup whole wheat bread crumbs

1 shallot, minced

1 garlic clove, minced

1 teaspoon grated lemon zest

½ teaspoon dried tarragon

Salt and black pepper (optional)

1 (16-ounce / 454-g) package sprouted or extra-firm tofu, drained and sliced lengthwise into 8 pieces

1 tablespoon Dijon mustard

1 tablespoon lemon juice

1. Preheat the oven to 375ºF (190ºC) and line a baking sheet with parchment paper. 2. Chop the pistachios in a food processor or with a knife until they are breadcrumb-sized. In a pie plate, mix them with bread crumbs, shallot, garlic, lemon zest, and tarragon. Season with salt and pepper if desired. 3. Season the tofu with salt and pepper. In a small bowl, combine mustard and lemon juice. 4. Spread the mustard mixture evenly over the top and sides of the tofu, then press each slice into the bread crumb mixture. 5. Place the tofu uncoated side down on the baking sheet. Sprinkle any leftover bread crumb mixture evenly on top. Bake until the tops are browned, about 20 minutes. Serve and enjoy your Nut-Crusted Tofu!

Per Serving: (1 slice)

calories: 114 | fat: 7g | protein: 8g | carbs: 7g | fiber: 1g

Curried Chickpeas and Rice

Prep time: 10 minutes | Cook time: 35 minutes | Serves 4

1 cup brown basmati rice ¼ cup finely chopped green scallions ¼ teaspoons cumin seeds, toasted ¼ teaspoons curry powder	½ teaspoons salt, or to taste (optional) 1½ cups cooked chickpeas ½ tablespoon fresh lime juice

1. Rinse the rice and cook it in a pot with 2½ cups of water. Bring to a boil, then simmer covered for 30 minutes until tender. 2. In a separate saucepan, cook scallions in 2 tablespoons of water until soft. Add cumin seeds, curry powder, salt (if desired), and chickpeas. Cook for a minute, then add the cooked rice and lime juice. Cook for another minute and serve hot. Enjoy your flavorful Curried Chickpeas and Rice!

Per Serving:

calories: 275 | fat: 3g | protein: 9g | carbs: 53g | fiber: 6g

Mushroom Barley Risotto

Prep time: 20 minutes | Cook time: 55 minutes | Serves 3 to 4

1 ounce (28 g) dried porcini mushrooms, soaked for 30 minutes in 1 cup of water that has just been boiled 3 large shallots, peeled and finely diced 8 ounces (227 g) cremini mushrooms, sliced 2 sage leaves, minced 3 cloves garlic, peeled and	minced 1½ cups pearled barley ½ cup dry white wine 3 to 4 cups vegetable stock, or low-sodium vegetable broth ¼ cup nutritional yeast (optional) Salt and freshly ground black pepper, to taste

1. Drain the porcini mushrooms, reserving the liquid, and finely chop them. 2. In a saucepan, sauté shallots over medium heat, adding water as needed. Add cremini mushrooms and cook until browned. Stir in sage, garlic, barley, and white wine for 1 minute. Add vegetable stock and porcini soaking liquid, bringing it to a boil. 3. Reduce heat and cook, covered, for 25 minutes. Add more broth if needed and cook for another 15 to 20 minutes. Stir in chopped porcini mushrooms and nutritional yeast (if desired). Season with salt and pepper, then serve your delicious Mushroom Barley Risotto immediately. Enjoy!

Per Serving:

calories: 354 | fat: 2g | protein: 15g | carbs: 74g | fiber: 16g

Barley Bowl with Cranberries and Walnuts

Prep time: 5 minutes | Cook time: 30 minutes | Serves 4

1 cup pearl barley, uncooked 3 cups water ¼ cup poppy seeds	½ cup dried cranberries ½ cup chopped walnuts, toasted

1. In a medium pot, boil the barley in water until tender (25 to 30 minutes). Drain any excess water and let it cool. 2. In a small bowl, soak poppy seeds and dried cranberries in hot water for 5 to 10 minutes, then drain and let cool. 3. In a large bowl, combine cooked barley, cranberries, poppy seeds, and walnuts. Mix well, cover, and refrigerate for 30 minutes to 1 hour before serving cold. Enjoy your delicious Barley Bowl!

Per Serving:

calories: 341 | fat: 14g | protein: 9g | carbs: 50g | fiber: 11g

Peanut Butter Tempeh

Prep time: 10 minutes | Cook time: 30 minutes | Serves 4

2 (8-ounce / 227-g) packages tempeh ½ cup creamy or crunchy peanut butter ⅓ cup nutritional yeast 1 tablespoon fresh lemon juice or apple cider vinegar	1 tablespoon reduced-sodium, gluten-free tamari ½ teaspoon black pepper ¼ teaspoon salt (optional) ⅛ teaspoon cayenne pepper ⅓ to ½ cup warm water

1. Preheat the oven to 375°F (190°C). Line a baking sheet with parchment paper. 2. Slice each block of tempeh into 8 pieces. Smash each one slightly with the heel of your hand to increase the surface area. 3. In a shallow dish, combine the peanut butter, nutritional yeast, lemon juice, tamari, pepper, salt (if desired), and cayenne with enough water to form a thick sauce. The sauce should be lighter in color than peanut butter and be thinner than ketchup. If it's too thick, add water, 1 tablespoon at a time. If it gets too thin, whisk in another tablespoon or two of peanut butter. 4. Coat each piece of tempeh with the sauce and place on the prepared baking sheet. Spoon any remaining sauce on top of the tempeh slices. 5. Bake for 15 minutes, flip the tempeh, if desired, then bake for another 15 minutes, or until the sauce has formed a crust on the tempeh and turned medium brown. Serve.

Per Serving:

calories: 369 | fat: 24g | protein: 25g | carbs: 19g | fiber: 5g

Texas Caviar

Prep time: 20 minutes | Cook time: 0 minutes | Serves 4

2½ cups cooked black-eyed peas	and minced
3 ears corn, kernels removed (about 2 cups)	½ cup finely chopped cilantro
1 medium ripe tomato, diced	¼ cup plus 2 tablespoons balsamic vinegar
½ medium red onion, peeled and diced small	3 cloves garlic, peeled and minced
½ red bell pepper, seeded and diced small	1 teaspoon cumin seeds, toasted and ground
1 jalapeño pepper, seeded	Salt, to taste (optional)

1. Mix all ingredients in a large bowl and refrigerate until well chilled, about 1 hour.

Per Serving:

calories: 165 | fat: 1g | protein: 7g | carbs: 34g | fiber: 6g

Red Peppers with Herby Breadcrumbs

Prep time: 10 minutes | Cook time: 40 minutes | Serves 6

4 red bell peppers, cores and stems removed	2 teaspoons minced fresh thyme leaves
3 tablespoons virgin olive oil, divided (optional)	1 clove garlic, minced
Salt and pepper, to taste (optional)	½ teaspoon fresh lemon zest
	¼ teaspoon nutritional yeast
2½ cups cubed stale bread	¼ cup chopped fresh flat-leaf parsley

1. Preheat the oven to 400°F (205°C). Line a baking sheet with parchment paper. 2. Cut each bell pepper into 4 segments. Remove any white pith pieces from the center, and place them on the baking sheet. Toss the bell peppers with 1 tablespoon of the olive oil, if using. Spread the peppers out into a single layer, and season with salt and pepper, if using. Slide the peppers into the oven, and roast until just tender, about 25 minutes. 3. Place the cubed bread into a food processor, and pulse the machine to make coarse crumbs. 4. Heat the remaining 2 tablespoons of the olive oil in a medium sauté pan over medium heat. Add the breadcrumbs to the pan along with some salt and pepper, if using. Cook the breadcrumbs, stirring frequently, until evenly golden brown, about 10 minutes. Add the thyme, garlic, lemon zest, and nutritional yeast, and cook until fragrant, about 30 seconds. 5. Remove the breadcrumbs from the heat, and stir in the chopped parsley. 6. Arrange the roasted peppers on a platter and shower with the warm breadcrumbs. Serve warm.

Per Serving:

calories: 252 | fat: 9g | protein: 7g | carbs: 36g | fiber: 3g

Black Bean and Quinoa Burrito Bowls

Prep time: 10 minutes | Cook time: 10 minutes | Serves 4

1 cup quinoa	½ teaspoon onion powder
1 cup frozen corn	½ teaspoon garlic powder
1 teaspoon extra-virgin olive oil (optional)	1 avocado, peeled, pitted, and sliced, for serving
1 tablespoon tomato paste	Shredded red cabbage, for serving
½ teaspoon salt, divided (optional)	Store-bought salsa, for serving
2¼ cups water	¼ cup chopped fresh cilantro, for garnish
1 (15-ounce / 425-g) can black beans	

1. In a medium saucepan over medium-high heat, combine the quinoa, corn, oil, tomato paste, ¼ teaspoon of salt (if using), and the water and bring it to a boil. Cover, lower the heat to low, and cook until the quinoa is tender and the water is absorbed, about 15 minutes. 2. In a skillet over medium heat, combine the black beans, onion powder, garlic powder, and the remaining ¼ teaspoon salt and cook, stirring, for 5 minutes. 3. To assemble, divide the quinoa mixture, black beans, avocado, cabbage, and salsa among 4 bowls. Garnish with the cilantro.

Per Serving:

calories: 379 | fat: 12g | protein: 14g | carbs: 58g | fiber: 13g

Orange Quinoa with Black Beans

Prep time: 15 minutes | Cook time: 20 minutes | Serves 4

1½ cups quinoa, rinsed and drained	2 tablespoons balsamic vinegar
1½ teaspoons cumin seeds, toasted and ground	Zest and juice of 1 orange (about ¼ cup juice)
2 cups cooked black beans, or 1 (15-ounce / 425-g) can, drained and rinsed	4 green onions (white and green parts), thinly sliced
	Salt and freshly ground black pepper, to taste
1½ teaspoons grated ginger	

1. Add 3 cups of water to a medium pot with a tight-fitting lid and bring to a boil over high heat. Add the quinoa and return the pot to a boil over high heat. Reduce the heat to medium-low and cook the quinoa, covered, for 15 to 20 minutes, or until tender. 2. Place the quinoa in a large bowl and add the cumin, black beans, ginger, vinegar, orange zest and juice, and green onions. Mix well and season with salt and pepper.

Per Serving:

calories: 369 | fat: 4g | protein: 16g | carbs: 65g | fiber: 12g

Cabbage and Millet Pilaf

Prep time: 15 minutes | Cook time: 45 minutes | Serves 4

2¼ cups vegetable stock, or low-sodium vegetable broth	1 celery stalk, diced
¾ cup millet	2 cloves garlic, peeled and minced
1 medium leek (white and light green parts), diced and rinsed	1 teaspoon minced thyme
	1 tablespoon minced dill
1 medium carrot, peeled and diced	3 cups chopped cabbage
	Salt and freshly ground black pepper, to taste

1. In a medium saucepan, bring the vegetable stock to a boil over high heat. Add the millet and bring the pot back to a boil over high heat. Reduce the heat to medium and cook, covered, for 20 minutes, or until the millet is tender and all the vegetable stock is absorbed. 2. Place the leek, carrot, and celery in a large saucepan and sauté over medium heat for 7 to 8 minutes. Add water 1 to 2 tablespoons at a time to keep the vegetables from sticking to the pan. Add the garlic, thyme, dill, and cabbage and cook, stirring frequently, over medium heat until the cabbage is tender, about 10 minutes. Add the cooked millet and cook for another 5 minutes, stirring frequently. Season with salt and pepper.

Per Serving:
calories: 193 | fat: 2g | protein: 5g | carbs: 39g | fiber: 6g

Lentil-Mushroom No-Meat Pasta (Bolognese)

Prep time: 15 minutes | Cook time: 45 minutes | Serves 4

¼ cup mushroom stock	1 cup brown lentils
1 large yellow onion, finely diced	1 (28-ounce / 794-g) can puréed or diced tomatoes with basil
1 (10-ounce / 283-g) package cremini mushrooms, trimmed and chopped fine	1 tablespoon balsamic vinegar
	Pasta
2 tablespoons tomato paste	Salt and black pepper (optional)
3 chopped garlic cloves	
1 teaspoon oregano	Chopped basil
2½ cups water	

1. Place a large stockpot over medium heat. Add the stock. Once the broth starts to simmer, add the onion and mushrooms. Cover and cook until both are soft, about 5 minutes. Add the tomato paste, garlic, and oregano and cook 2 minutes, stirring constantly. 2. Stir in the water and lentils. Bring to a boil, then reduce the heat to medium-low and cook for 5 minutes, covered. Add the tomatoes and vinegar. Replace the lid, reduce the heat to low and cook until the lentils are tender, about 30 minutes. 3. Meanwhile, cook the pasta according to the package instructions. 4. Remove the sauce

from the heat and season with salt (if desired) and pepper to taste. Garnish with the basil and serve atop the pasta.

Per Serving:
calories: 181 | fat: 1g | protein: 9g | carbs: 40g | fiber: 7g

Quick Panfried Tempeh

Prep time: 5 minutes | Cook time: 10 minutes | Serves 2

2 tablespoons extra-virgin coconut oil, plus more as needed (optional)	into ¼-inch slices
	Flaky or fine sea salt (optional)
½ pound (227 g) tempeh, cut	

1. Warm a large skillet over medium heat and add coconut oil, tilting the pan to coat. 2. Add sliced tempeh in a single layer and cook until golden, about 3 to 4 minutes. 3. Flip the tempeh and cook the other side until golden and crisp, adding more oil if needed. 4. Repeat with any remaining tempeh, adding more oil before adding the slices. 5. Transfer the cooked tempeh to a serving plate, sprinkle with salt, and serve warm. Enjoy your delicious panfried tempeh!

Per Serving:
calories: 336 | fat: 25g | protein: 2g | carbs: 11g | fiber: 0g

Chorizo Chickpea Bowl

Prep time: 10 minutes | Cook time: 10 minutes | Serves 4

2 cups cooked or canned chickpeas	chorizo seasoning
	½ cup water
1 cup fresh or frozen spinach	Optional Toppings:
¼ cup raisins	Raisins
½ cup raw and unsalted cashews	Parsley
	Lime juice
2 tablespoons Mexican	

1. When using dry chickpeas, soak and cook ⅔ cup of dry chickpeas. 2. Put a nonstick deep frying pan over medium-high heat and add the spinach, chorizo seasoning and the water. 3. Stir continuously until everything is cooked, then add the chickpeas and cashew nuts. Make sure to stir again to mix everything. 4. Let it cook for about 10 minutes while stirring occasionally. 5. Turn the heat off, then add the raisins, stir well and drain the excess water. 6. Divide between 2 bowls, garnish with the optional toppings, serve and enjoy! 7. Store the chorizo chickpeas in an airtight container in the fridge, and consume within 2 days. Alternatively, store in the freezer for a maximum of 30 days and thaw at room temperature. The chorizo chickpeas can be eaten cold or reheated in a saucepan or a microwave.

Per Serving:
calories: 307 | fat: 10g | protein: 14g | carbs: 41g | fiber: 11g

Thai-Inspired Rice Bowl

Prep time: 30 minutes | Cook time: 45 minutes | Serves 4

Peanut Sauce:	1 small red cabbage, shredded
3 tablespoons creamy peanut butter	1 red bell pepper, cut into slices
2 tablespoons freshly squeezed lime juice	1 yellow bell pepper, cut into slices
1 tablespoon packed lime zest	1 cup shelled edamame
1 tablespoon coconut aminos	1 shallot, cut into slices
1 tablespoon grated peeled fresh ginger	1 carrot, cut into matchsticks
2 garlic cloves, minced	¼ cup fresh cilantro, chopped
½ teaspoon red pepper flakes	1 bunch chopped scallions, green parts only
Rice Bowl:	Juice of 1 lime
1½ cups water	
¾ cup brown rice	

Make the Peanut Sauce: 1. In a medium bowl, whisk together the peanut butter, lime juice and zest, coconut aminos, ginger, garlic, and red pepper flakes to combine. Set aside. Make the Rice Bowl: 2. In a medium pot over high heat, bring the water to a boil. Stir in the brown rice. Bring to a simmer, reduce the heat to medium-low, cover the pot, and cook, undisturbed, for 35 to 40 minutes. Check the rice after 35 minutes to see if the water has been absorbed. Remove from the heat. 3. In a large bowl, toss together the brown rice, red cabbage, red and yellow bell peppers, edamame, shallot, carrot, cilantro, scallions, and lime juice. Serve with a drizzle of peanut sauce.

Per Serving:

calories: 323 | fat: 9g | protein: 14g | carbs: 54g | fiber: 11g

Butter Bean Pâté

Prep time: 15 minutes | Cook time: 0 minutes | Serves 4

3 cups cooked butter beans or 2 (15½-ounce /439-g) cans beans, drained and well rinsed	½ teaspoon finely grated or pressed garlic
¼ cup extra-virgin olive oil (optional)	½ teaspoon fine sea salt, or more to taste (optional)
	Freshly ground black pepper

1. Put the beans, olive oil, garlic, salt, if using, and pepper in a food processor and process until completely smooth, with a fluffy whipped texture; this will take a couple of minutes to achieve. Season to taste with more salt and pepper if necessary. Serve, or store in an airtight container in the fridge for up to 4 days.

Per Serving:

calories: 253 | fat: 15g | protein: 9g | carbs: 23g | fiber: 8g

Pasta Marinara with Spicy Italian Bean Balls

Prep time: 20 minutes | Cook time: 35 minutes | Serves 4

Spicy Italian Bean Balls:	½ cup whole-grain bread crumbs
¼ cup vegetable broth	Weeknight Marinara:
½ yellow onion, minced	2 tablespoons mushroom stock
2 teaspoons dried oregano	Handful basil leaves
1 teaspoon fennel seeds	3 garlic cloves, minced
1 teaspoon garlic powder	1 (28-ounce / 794-g) can whole tomatoes with juice reserved
½ teaspoon crushed red pepper	Salt (optional)
1 (15-ounce / 425-g) can white beans, drained and rinsed	Pasta
Salt and black pepper (optional)	

1. To make the bean balls, preheat the oven to 350ºF (180ºC). Line a baking sheet with parchment paper. 2. Heat a medium skillet over medium heat, then add the broth. Add the onion and cook, stirring often, until it begins to soften, about 5 minutes. 3. Add the oregano, fennel seeds, garlic powder, and crushed red pepper. Cook until fragrant, about 1 minute longer. Remove from the heat and transfer to a food processor along with the beans. 4. Pulse to combine and season with salt (if desired) and pepper to taste; add the bread crumbs. Pulse until just combined. 5. Using a 2-ounce (57-g) cookie scoop, form balls (it may be necessary to wet hands to prevent sticking). Bake for 15 minutes, flip, and bake 15 minutes longer, or until golden brown. 6. Meanwhile, make the marinara: Place a medium saucepan over medium-high heat. Add the stock to the hot pan. Once it's warm, add the basil and garlic and cook for 2 minutes, stirring occasionally. Stir in the tomatoes with their juice, bring just to a boil, then reduce heat to low, cover, and cook for 15 minutes. Season with salt, if desired. 7. Cook the pasta according to package instructions. Serve topped with the bean balls.

Per Serving:

calories: 311 | fat: 3g | protein: 16g | carbs: 58g | fiber: 12g

Chapter 6 Snacks and Appetizers

Chocolate Trail Mix Bars

Prep time: 30 minutes | Cook time: 0 minutes | Makes 8 bars

¾ cup old-fashioned oats
½ cup bran flakes cereal
½ cup chopped mixed nuts
¼ cup dried cherries
¼ cup dried cranberries

¼ cup raw shelled hempseed
3 tablespoons peanut butter
¼ cup maple syrup (optional)
½ cup melted dairy-free chocolate chips

1. Line an 8-inch square baking dish with parchment paper, leaving handles on opposite sides for easy removal. 2. In a large bowl, combine oats, cereal, nuts, cherries, cranberries, and hempseed. Mix well. 3. Mix peanut butter and syrup together, then add to the bowl. Stir to combine. Add melted chocolate and mix again. 4. Press mixture firmly into the prepared dish and refrigerate for 30 minutes to set. 5. Lift the bars using the parchment paper handles, place on a cutting board, and slice into eight bars.

Per Serving: (1 bar)

calories: 169 | fat: 9g | protein: 16g | carbs: 19g | fiber: 3g

Tempeh Stuffed Cremini Mushrooms

Prep time: 15 minutes | Cook time: 40 minutes | Serves 6

18 cremini mushrooms
2 tablespoons diced red onion, small dice
3 ounces (85 g) tempeh, diced very small, or pulsed

small
Pinch of onion powder
Pinch of cayenne pepper
¼ cup rice, cooked
1 tablespoon tamari

1. Remove stems from mushrooms and finely chop them. Set mushroom caps aside. 2. Sauté chopped stems and onion in water for 10-15 minutes until onion is translucent. Add tempeh and cook for 5 more minutes. Stir in onion powder, cayenne pepper, rice, and tamari, and cook for 2 more minutes. 3. Preheat oven to 350°F (180°C). 4. Stuff mushroom caps with the mixture and place on a baking sheet. Bake for 20 minutes.

Per Serving: (3 mushrooms)

calories: 58 | fat: 3g | protein: 6g | carbs: 6g | fiber: 2g

Chewy Almond Butter Balls

Prep time: 15 minutes | Cook time: 0 minutes | Serves 2

2 tablespoons maple syrup (optional)
½ cup vanilla or chocolate flavor vegan protein powder
¼ cup almond butter

1 tablespoon pure vanilla extract
1 cup puffy rice cereal
1 tablespoon carob chips

1. In a large bowl, mix together maple syrup (if desired), protein powder, almond butter, and vanilla. Microwave the bowl for about 40 seconds until the ingredients are heated and the syrup and butter are melted. Add puffy rice cereal and carob chips, stirring everything evenly. 2. Line a sheet pan with parchment paper. Using a spoon, scoop out the mixture and shape it into small-to-medium sized balls with your hands, pressing firmly to prevent crumbling. Place the balls on the parchment paper-lined pan. Freeze for about 1 hour or refrigerate for 4 hours. 3. Enjoy the chewy almond butter balls cold or at room temperature. Store them in a container or Ziploc bag for later enjoyment.

Per Serving:

calories: 329 | fat: 16g | protein: 20g | carbs: 25g | fiber: 1g

Tropical Lemon Protein Bites

Prep time: 20 minutes | Cook time: 0 minutes | Makes 24 balls

1¾ cups cashews
¼ cup coconut flour
¼ cup unsweetened shredded coconut
3 tablespoons raw shelled

hempseed
3 tablespoons maple syrup (optional)
3 tablespoons fresh lemon juice

1. Add cashews to a food processor and process until finely ground. Then, add all the other ingredients to the food processor and blend until well combined. Transfer the mixture to a large bowl. 2. Take a portion of the dough and press it together with your hands to form a ball. Repeat this process until all the mixture is shaped into balls. Enjoy these delightful and nutritious protein bites with a tropical lemon flavor!

Per Serving: (2 balls)

calories: 165 | fat: 9g | protein: 8g | carbs: 13g | fiber: 1g

Carrot Cake Two-Bite Balls

Prep time: 20 minutes | Cook time: 0 minutes | Makes 16 balls

1 cup old-fashioned oats	15 dates, pitted
½ cup almond meal	2 tablespoons unsweetened
½ cup pecans	cocoa powder
⅓ cup plus 2 tablespoons	2 tablespoons almond butter
unsweetened shredded	1 teaspoon ground cinnamon
coconut, divided	½ teaspoon ground nutmeg
3 grated medium carrots	½ teaspoon ground ginger

1. In a food processor, combine oats, almond meal, pecans, ⅓ cup coconut, carrots, dates, and cocoa powder. Process on high until well mixed, scraping down the edges if needed. Add almond butter, cinnamon, nutmeg, and ginger, and mix again until well combined. 2. Transfer the mixture to a flat surface and ensure it's well blended. Use your hands if necessary. Pinch off pieces of dough and roll them into sixteen balls. Optionally, roll the balls in additional shredded coconut. Enjoy your delicious Carrot Cake Two-Bite Balls!

Per Serving: (2 balls)

calories: 194 | fat: 12g | protein: 8g | carbs: 24g | fiber: 6g

Protein Power Grilled Veggie and Fruit Skewers

Prep time: 15 minutes | Cook time: 25 minutes | Serves 4

8 ounces (227 g) extra-firm tofu, drained, pressed, and cut into 1-inch cubes	4 ounces (113 g) cremini mushrooms
2 tablespoons tamari	1 pineapple, chopped into chunks
1 tablespoon rice vinegar	1 red bell pepper, chopped into large pieces
1 tablespoon maple syrup (optional)	1 yellow bell pepper, chopped into large pieces
¼ teaspoon chili powder	Extra virgin olive oil, for grilling (optional)
1 large sweet potato, peeled and chopped into bite-size chunks	

1. Prepare the peppers by cutting off the stem end, slicing them lengthwise, and removing any seeds. Set aside. 2. In a food processor, combine all the remaining ingredients and pulse four or five times, leaving the chickpeas chunky. Stir the mixture to ensure it's well-blended. 3. Stuff each pepper half with approximately 2 tablespoons of the chickpea mixture. Set the stuffed peppers on a plate and serve. Now, you have your delicious Protein Power Grilled Veggie and Fruit Skewers ready to enjoy!

Per Serving: (2 skewers)

calories: 236 | fat: 4g | protein: 16g | carbs: 45g | fiber: 6g

Chocolate Cake Munch Cookies

Prep time: 10 minutes | Cook time: 10 minutes | Serves 12

½ cup dairy-free butter, softened	2 cups whole wheat flour
1 cup coconut sugar (optional)	¼ cup protein powder
1 tablespoon chia seeds or ground chia seeds	1 teaspoon baking powder
¾ cup soy milk	½ teaspoon baking soda
1 teaspoon vanilla	½ teaspoon salt (optional)
	½ cup cocoa powder
	1 cup chopped walnuts

1. In a stand mixer, combine butter and sugar (if using) and mix on medium speed for 5 minutes. 2. Mix chia seeds with 3 tablespoons of water. 3. Add chia mixture, milk, and vanilla to the butter and mix well at medium speed. 4. In a separate medium bowl, combine flour, protein powder, baking powder, baking soda, salt (if using), and cocoa, and mix well. 5. Turn mixer to medium and slowly add the dry mixture. Add walnuts and mix at low speed until combined. Refrigerate the mixture for 1 hour to overnight. 6. Preheat the oven to 400ºF (205ºC) and line a baking sheet with parchment paper. 7. Drop heaping tablespoons of dough onto the prepared cookie sheet, 2 inches apart. Roll into balls and then flatten by about half using the bottom of a measuring cup or other sturdy object. 8. Bake for 8 minutes, then cool on a wire rack. Enjoy your delicious Chocolate Cake Munch Cookies!

Per Serving: (2 cookies)

calories: 239 | fat: 16g | protein: 7g | carbs: 21g | fiber: 4g

Rainbow Veggie Protein Pinwheels

Prep time: 20 minutes | Cook time: 0 minutes | Serves 6

¼ cup hummus	¼ cup thinly sliced yellow bell pepper
¼ cup tempeh, crumbled in a food processor	1 thinly sliced carrot
2 large spinach tortillas	¼ cup thinly sliced purple cabbage
¼ cup thinly sliced red bell pepper	

1. Mix hummus and tempeh together. 2. Lay out tortillas and spread a thin layer of the hummus mixture on each tortilla, leaving a 1-inch border. Place thin strips of each vegetable next to each other over the hummus. 3. Roll the tortillas tightly and cut crosswise into pinwheels. The hummus will help them stick together at the edges. Enjoy your colorful and delicious Rainbow Veggie Protein Pinwheels!

Per Serving: (2 pinwheels)

calories: 66 | fat: 2g | protein: 9g | carbs: 8g | fiber: 4g

Strawberry-Avocado Toast with Balsamic Glaze

Prep time: 5 minutes | Cook time: 0 minute | Serves 2

1 avocado, peeled, pitted, and quartered	4 ripe strawberries, cut into ¼-inch slices
4 whole-wheat bread slices, toasted	1 tablespoon balsamic glaze or reduction

1. Mash one-quarter of the avocado on a slice of toast. 2. Layer one-quarter of the strawberry slices over the avocado. 3. Finish with a drizzle of balsamic glaze. 4. Repeat with the remaining ingredients and serve. Enjoy!

Per Serving:

calories: 150 | fat: 8g | protein: 5g | carbs: 17g | fiber: 5g

Kale Chips

Prep time: 5 minutes | Cook time: 20 minutes | Serves 4

¼ cup vegetable broth	½ teaspoon onion powder
1 tablespoon nutritional yeast	6 ounces (170 g) kale, stemmed and cut into 2- to 3-inch pieces
½ teaspoon garlic powder	

1. Preheat the oven to 300ºF (150ºC) and line a baking sheet with parchment paper. 2. In a small bowl, mix together the broth, nutritional yeast, garlic powder, and onion powder. 3. Put the kale in a large bowl and pour the seasoned broth over it. Toss well to coat the kale thoroughly. 4. Arrange the kale pieces in an even layer on the baking sheet. Bake for 20 minutes, turning the kale halfway through, until crispy. Enjoy your delicious homemade Kale Chips!

Per Serving:

calories: 41 | fat: 0g | protein: 4g | carbs: 7g | fiber: 2g

Avomame Spread

Prep time: 10 minutes | Cook time: 0 minutes | Makes 1½ cups

1 cup frozen shelled edamame beans, thawed	1 teaspoon grated fresh ginger
1 tablespoon apple cider vinegar, or lemon juice, or lime juice	1 avocado, coarsely chopped
1 tablespoon tamari or soy sauce	¼ cup fresh cilantro, basil, mint, or parsley, chopped
	½ cup alfalfa sprouts (optional)

1. In a food processor, pulse the beans with a bit of water and apple cider vinegar until they are roughly chopped. If you don't have a food processor, you can thaw the beans and chop them manually. 2. Add tamari, ginger, and avocado to the processor and puree until well combined. Then add cilantro and sprouts (if using) and puree again until smooth. If you don't have a food processor, mash the avocado and finely chop the remaining ingredients, then mix them together until well blended.

Per Serving:

calories: 265 | fat: 18g | protein: 11g | carbs: 17g | fiber: 11g

Greens and Beans Dip

Prep time: 10 minutes | Cook time: 0 minutes | Makes about 2 cups

1 (14-ounce / 397-g) can white beans, drained and rinsed, or 1½ cups cooked	1 tablespoon nutritional yeast (optional)
Zest and juice of 1 lemon	1 to 2 teaspoons curry powder
1 tablespoon almond butter, tahini, or other mild nut or seed butter	1 to 2 teaspoons ground cumin
1 to 2 leaves kale, rinsed and stemmed	1 teaspoon smoked paprika
	¼ teaspoon sea salt (optional)

1. Place all the ingredients in a food processor and pulse until they form a cohesive mixture. If you don't have a food processor, mash the beans and chop the kale separately, then combine them. 2. Taste the dip and adjust the seasoning to your liking, adding more spices, lemon juice, or salt (if using) as desired. Enjoy this flavorful dip with your favorite chips, crackers, or veggies!

Per Serving: (1 cup)

calories: 112 | fat: 5g | protein: 6g | carbs: 13g | fiber: 6g

Legit Salsa

Prep time: 10 minutes | Cook time: 0 minutes | Makes 5 cups

2 jalapeño chile peppers, diced	2 garlic cloves, halved
1 yellow onion, quartered	1 (28-ounce / 794-g) can diced tomatoes, undrained
1 small bunch fresh cilantro, leaves and tender stems	¼ cup fresh lime juice
	1 teaspoon sea salt (optional)

1. In a blender, combine all the ingredients and pulse until you achieve your preferred texture. Taste and add more salt (if using) as needed. 2. Transfer the salsa to an airtight container and store it in the refrigerator for up to 1 week. Enjoy the flavorful salsa with your favorite dishes!

Per Serving:

calories: 43 | fat: 0g | protein: 2g | carbs: 9g | fiber: 4g

Gingerbread Protein Bars

Prep time: 20 minutes | Cook time: 15 minutes | Makes 8 bars

2 cups raw and unsalted almonds	chocolate flavor
10 pitted dates	1 (4-inch) piece ginger, minced
4 tablespoons five-spice powder	Optional Toppings:
2 scoops soy protein isolate,	Cocoa powder
	Shredded coconut

1. Preheat the oven to 257°F (125°C) and roast almonds on a baking sheet for 10 to 15 minutes. 2. Soak dates in water for 10 minutes, then drain. 3. Blend almonds, dates, 5-spice powder, protein powder, and ginger in a food processor. 4. Line a loaf pan with parchment paper, add the mixture, and press it down firmly. 5. Chill the pan in the fridge for 45 minutes to firm up. 6. Divide into 8 bars, serve cold with optional toppings, and enjoy! 7. Store the bars in an airtight container in the fridge for up to 6 days or freeze for up to 90 days.

Per Serving:

calories: 263 | fat: 18g | protein: 16g | carbs: 9g | fiber: 4g

Popeye Protein Balls

Prep time: 5 minutes | Cook time: 0 minutes | Makes 20 to 26 balls

1 cup raw hazelnuts	powder
¼ cup pumpkin seeds	1 teaspoon ground cinnamon
Handful of fresh baby spinach	Pinch of Himalayan pink salt (optional)
2 tablespoons raw cacao or carob powder	2 to 4 tablespoons superfood powder (açaí, maqui,
1 cup raisins, soaked in water for 15 minutes, rinsed and drained	maca, spirulina, matcha or moringa), depending on potency, for dusting
2 tablespoons hemp protein	(optional)

1. In a food processor with the S blade, combine all ingredients except the superfood powder. Process until a ball forms, being careful not to overprocess. If the mixture becomes too soft, add up to 2 tablespoons of pumpkin seeds and refrigerate for 30 minutes before forming into balls. 2. Shape the mixture into balls using a tablespoon or your hands. Roll between your palms. 3. Place the balls on a plate and refrigerate for at least 1 hour before serving. 4. Optionally, before refrigerating, roll the balls in a plate of superfood powder to coat the exterior. Enjoy!

Per Serving:

calories: 167 | fat: 10g | protein: 5g | carbs: 15g | fiber: 2g

Hazelnut Choco Plum Bites

Prep time: 45 minutes | Cook time: 0 minutes | Makes 12 balls

2 cups roasted hazelnuts	½ cup cocoa powder
8 dried pitted plums	Optional Toppings:
1 cup soy protein isolate, chocolate flavor	Crushed dark chocolate
	Crushed hazelnuts

1. Transfer hazelnuts, plums, and soy protein isolate to a food processor and blend into a smooth mixture. Alternatively, use a medium bowl and a handheld blender. 2. Line a baking sheet with parchment paper. 3. Scoop out a heaping tablespoon of the chocolate hazelnut mixture and roll it into a firm ball using your hands. Repeat for the other 11 balls. 4. Place cocoa powder in a medium bowl and roll the balls in it, then transfer them to the baking sheet. 5. Refrigerate the baking sheet for about 45 minutes until the balls firm up. 6. Serve the hazelnut chocolate balls right away with optional toppings or store them in an airtight container in the fridge for up to 6 days. Alternatively, store in the freezer in Ziploc bags for up to 90 days and thaw at room temperature. Enjoy!

Per Serving:

calories: 169 | fat: 11g | protein: 10g | carbs: 7g | fiber: 4g

Choco Almond Bars

Prep time: 10 minutes | Cook time: 15 minutes | Makes 4 bars

1 cup raw and unsalted almonds	chocolate flavor
5 pitted dates	Optional Toppings:
1 scoop soy protein isolate,	Shredded coconut
	Cocoa powder

1. Preheat the oven to 257°F (125°C) and line a baking sheet with parchment paper. 2. Put the almonds on the baking sheet and roast them for about 10 to 15 minutes or until they're fragrant. 3. Meanwhile, cover the dates with water in a small bowl and let them sit for about 10 minutes. Drain the dates after soaking and make sure no water is left. 4. Take the almonds out of the oven and let them cool down for about 5 minutes. 5. Add all the ingredients to a food processor and blend into a chunky mixture. 6. Alternatively, add all ingredients to a medium bowl, cover it, and process using a handheld blender. 7. Line a loaf pan with parchment paper. Add the almond mixture to the loaf pan, spread it out and press it down firmly until it is 1 inch (2.5 cm) thick all over. 8. Divide into 4 bars, serve cold with the optional toppings and enjoy! 9. Store the bars in an airtight container in the fridge and consume within 4 days. Alternatively, store in the freezer for a maximum of 90 days and thaw at room temperature.

Per Serving:

calories: 254 | fat: 18g | protein: 16g | carbs: 8g | fiber: 4g

Tempeh Chickpea Stuffed Mini Peppers

Prep time: 20 minutes | Cook time: 0 minutes | Serves 6

12 ounces (340 g) multi-colored sweet mini peppers	½ cup dairy-free mayonnaise
2 (15 ounces / 425 g) cans chickpeas, drained and rinsed	¼ cup cider vinegar
	1 teaspoon ground mustard
	3 scallions, thinly sliced
¾ cup tempeh, chopped	1 teaspoon salt (optional)
	¼ teaspoon cayenne pepper

1. Cut off the stem end of the peppers, slice them lengthwise, and remove any seeds inside. Set aside. 2. In a food processor, combine all the remaining ingredients and pulse a few times until the chickpeas are chunky. Remove the blade and stir to ensure the mixture is well blended. 3. Stuff each pepper half with about 2 tablespoons of the chickpea mixture. Place the stuffed peppers on a plate and serve. Enjoy these delicious Tempeh Chickpea Stuffed Mini Peppers!

Per Serving: (2 mini peppers)

calories: 231 | fat: 11g | protein: 10g | carbs: 25g | fiber: 6g

Lemon-Oatmeal Cacao Cookies

Prep time: 30 minutes | Cook time: 35 minutes | Makes 14 cookies

12 pitted Medjool dates	more as needed (optional)
Boiling water, for soaking the dates	1½ cups old-fashioned oats
1 cup unsweetened applesauce	1 cup oat flour
	¾ cup coarsely chopped walnuts
1 tablespoon freshly squeezed lemon juice	2 tablespoons lemon zest
1 teaspoon vanilla extract	1 tablespoon cacao powder
1 tablespoon water, plus	½ teaspoon baking soda

1. In a small bowl, soak dates in boiling water for 15 to 20 minutes to soften. 2. Preheat the oven to 300ºF (150ºC) and line 2 baking sheets with parchment paper or silicone mats. 3. Drain dates and blend them with applesauce, lemon juice, and vanilla until a thick paste forms. Add water if needed for smoothness. 4. In a large bowl, mix oats, oat flour, walnuts, lemon zest, cacao powder, and baking soda. Stir in the date mixture. 5. Scoop ¼-cup portions of dough, roll into balls, and press lightly on the baking sheets. Flatten to about 1 inch thick and 3 inches in diameter. 6. Bake for 30 to 35 minutes until cookies are crispy and dry on top. Cool on a wire rack. 7. Store the cookies in an airtight container at room temperature for up to 1 week. Enjoy your delightful Lemon-Oatmeal Cacao Cookies!

Per Serving: (1 cookie)

calories: 174 | fat: 6g | protein: 4g | carbs: 30g | fiber: 4g

Baked Vegetable Chips

Prep time: 20 minutes | Cook time: 35 minutes | Serves 2

1 pound (454 g) starchy root vegetables, such as russet potato, sweet potato, rutabaga, parsnip, red or golden beet, or taro	moisture
	1 teaspoon garlic powder
	1 teaspoon paprika
	½ teaspoon onion powder
1 pound (454 g) high-water vegetables, such as zucchini or summer squash	½ teaspoon freshly ground black pepper
	1 teaspoon avocado oil or other oil (optional)
Kosher salt, for absorbing	

1. Preheat the oven to 300ºF (150ºC) and line 2 baking sheets with parchment paper. 2. Scrub and wash the root vegetables and high-water vegetables. 3. Slice all vegetables into ⅛-inch-thick slices using a mandoline or sharp kitchen knife. 4. Sprinkle sliced high-water vegetables with kosher salt and let sit for 15 minutes to draw out moisture. Dab off excess moisture and salt. 5. In a small bowl, mix garlic powder, paprika, onion powder, and pepper. 6. Arrange the sliced vegetables on baking sheets in a single layer. Brush with oil, if desired, and sprinkle with the spice mix. 7. Bake for 35 minutes, switching the pans halfway through baking for even cooking. 8. Transfer the chips to a wire rack to cool and crisp. Enjoy your homemade vegetable chips!

Per Serving:

calories: 250 | fat: 3g | protein: 8g | carbs: 51g | fiber: 6g

Mocha Chocolate Brownie Bars

Prep time: 15 minutes | Cook time: 0 minutes | Serves 3

2½ cups chocolate or vanilla vegan protein powder	extract
	¼ teaspoon nutmeg
½ cup cocoa powder	2 tablespoons agave nectar (optional)
½ cup old-fashioned or quick oats	1 cup cold brewed coffee
1 teaspoon pure vanilla	

1. Line a square baking dish with parchment paper and set it aside. 2. In a large bowl, mix together the dry ingredients. Slowly add agave nectar (if desired), vanilla extract, and cold coffee while stirring constantly until the mixture becomes smooth and lump-free. Pour the batter into the prepared dish, pressing it into the corners. Refrigerate for about 4 hours until firm, or use the freezer for just 1 hour. 3. Once firm, slice the mixture into 6 even squares, and they're ready to enjoy, share, or store!

Per Serving:

calories: 213 | fat: 4g | protein: 27g | carbs: 17g | fiber: 4g

Roasted Taco-Seasoned Edamame and Chickpeas

Prep time: 10 minutes | Cook time: 30 minutes | Serves 7

12 ounces (340 g) frozen edamame	liquid to use as aquafaba) and rinsed
1 (15 ounces / 425 g) can chickpeas, drained (save the	4 tablespoons taco seasoning
	3 tablespoons aquafaba

1. Preheat the oven to 400°F (205°C). 2. Cook the edamame as directed on the package. 3. Spread chickpeas and cooked edamame on a baking sheet and bake for 20 minutes. 4. In a medium bowl, combine the taco seasoning. 5. Remove the edamame and chickpeas from the oven, toss with aquafaba, and coat with the taco seasoning mixture. 6. Return to the oven and bake for another 10 minutes. 7. Let them cool in the oven for at least 2 hours to overnight before storing in an airtight container. Enjoy! They will keep for 2 weeks.

Per Serving: (½ cup)

calories: 159 | fat: 4g | protein: 10g | carbs: 21g | fiber: 7g

No-Bake Chocolate Peanut Butter Cookies

Prep time: 20 minutes | Cook time: 5 minutes | Makes 24 cookies

½ cup unsweetened dairy-free milk	⅓ cup dairy-free semi-sweet chocolate chips
3 tablespoons dairy-free butter	1 teaspoon vanilla extract
⅓ cup coconut sugar (optional)	⅓ cup creamy peanut butter
1 tablespoon unsweetened cocoa powder	Pinch of salt (optional)
	2½ cups old-fashioned oats or quick-cooking oats
	¼ cup raw shelled hempseed

1. Line a baking sheet with wax paper. 2. Place the milk, butter, sugar (if desired), cocoa powder, and chocolate chips in a large saucepan. Bring to a rolling boil and then look at the timer. Let boil for 2 minutes. Stir occasionally so that the chocolate chips don't stick to the bottom of the pan before they melt. Remove from the heat and add the vanilla, peanut butter, and salt (if desired) and mix until the peanut butter melts. Stir in the oats and hempseed. 3. With a spoon, drop dollops of the batter onto the prepared baking sheet. Within a minute or less you can handle them and shape into cookies. Let the cookies set for an hour or so. You can speed up the cooling and hardening process by placing them in the refrigerator.

Per Serving: (2 cookies)

calories: 220 | fat: 77g | protein: 7g | carbs: 29g | fiber: 5g

Salsa with Mushrooms and Olives

Prep time: 30 minutes | Cook time: 0 minutes | Serves 3

½ cup finely chopped white button mushrooms	1 tablespoon finely chopped scallions
1 tablespoon chopped fresh parsley	⅓ cup chopped marinated artichoke hearts
1 tablespoon chopped fresh basil	½ cup chopped olives
2 Roma tomatoes, finely chopped	1 tablespoon balsamic vinegar
	3 slices sourdough toast

1. Combine mushrooms, parsley, basil, tomatoes, scallions, artichoke hearts, and olives in a medium mixing bowl. 2. Dress with balsamic vinegar and let marinate at room temperature for about 20 minutes or refrigerate until serving time. 3. Serve the salsa with slices of sourdough toast.

Per Serving:

calories: 205 | fat: 3g | protein: 9g | carbs: 41g | fiber: 4g

Homemade Popcorn with Magic Dust

Prep time: 10 minutes | Cook time: 10 minutes | Serves 8

⅓ cup raw cashews	½ teaspoon ground turmeric
2 tablespoons nutritional yeast	½ teaspoon garlic powder
1 tablespoon arrowroot powder	Freshly ground black pepper, to taste
2 teaspoons fine sea salt (optional)	¼ cup refined coconut oil (optional)
	⅔ cup organic popping corn

1. Process cashews, nutritional yeast, arrowroot powder, sea salt (if using), turmeric, garlic powder, and black pepper in a food processor to create the magic dust. Set aside. 2. Prepare a large bowl for the popped popcorn. 3. Heat coconut oil and 3 popcorn kernels in a pot over medium-high heat. Once the 3 kernels pop, remove them and add the rest of the popcorn kernels. Cover and wait for 30 seconds. 4. Return the pot to the heat and shake vigorously for about 2 minutes until popping slows. Remove from heat and remove the lid immediately. 5. Transfer the popcorn to the large bowl. Sprinkle ¾ of the magic dust and mix well with your hands. Garnish with the remaining magic dust and serve immediately.

Per Serving:

calories: 144 | fat: 12g | protein: 3g | carbs: 7g | fiber: 1g

Crispy Chickpea Snackers

Prep time: 10 minutes | Cook time: 4 to 6 hours | Makes 7 to 8 cups

4 (14½-ounce / 411-g) cans chickpeas, drained and rinsed Juice of 2 lemons	1 tablespoon garlic powder 1 tablespoon onion powder 2 teaspoons paprika Salt (optional)

1. Place the chickpeas in the slow cooker and add lemon juice, garlic powder, onion powder, and paprika. Season with salt (if using). Mix well to coat the chickpeas with seasoning. 2. Cover the slow cooker with a slightly open lid to allow steam to escape. Cook on High for 4 to 6 hours or on Low for 8 to 10 hours, stirring every 30 to 45 minutes to prevent burning. Enjoy the delicious Crispy Chickpea Snackers!

Per Serving:

calories: 56 | fat: 1g | protein: 3g | carbs: 9g | fiber: 3g

Protein Peanut Butter Balls

Prep time: 20 minutes | Cook time: 0 minutes | Makes 24 balls

½ cup creamy peanut butter ½ cup maple syrup (optional) ½ cup powdered soy milk, non-GMO	¼ cup flaxseed meal ½ cup coconut flour ¼ cup peanuts, chopped fine

1. In a medium bowl, mix together peanut butter and maple syrup (if desired). Add powdered soy milk, flaxseed meal, and coconut flour. Mix well and roll the mixture into 24 balls. Lightly roll each ball in chopped peanuts. 2. Store the Peanut Butter Balls in the refrigerator for up to 2 weeks. Enjoy your Protein Peanut Butter Balls!

Per Serving: (2 balls)

calories: 133 | fat: 8g | protein: 10g | carbs: 12g | fiber: 2g

Oat Crunch Apple Crisp

Prep time: 10 minutes | Cook time: 35 minutes | Serves 6

3 medium apples, cored and cut into ¼-inch pieces ¾ cup apple juice 1 teaspoon vanilla extract	1 teaspoon ground cinnamon, divided 2 cups rolled oats ¼ cup maple syrup (optional)

1. Preheat the oven to 375ºF (190ºC). 2. In a large bowl, mix together apple slices, apple juice, vanilla, and ½ teaspoon of cinnamon until the apple slices are coated. 3. Place the apple slices in the bottom of a round or square baking dish. Pour any leftover liquid over the apples. 4. In another bowl, combine oats, maple syrup (if desired), and the remaining ½ teaspoon of cinnamon, coating the oats evenly. 5. Sprinkle the oat mixture over the apples, ensuring even coverage. 6. Bake for 35 minutes, or until the oats turn golden brown. Serve this delicious Oat Crunch Apple Crisp and enjoy!

Per Serving:

calories: 213 | fat: 2g | protein: 4g | carbs: 47g | fiber: 6g

Olive-Chickpea Waffles

Prep time: 10 minutes | Cook time: 30 minutes | Makes 6 waffles

2 cups chickpea flour 1 tablespoon chopped rosemary or thyme 1 teaspoon gluten-free baking powder ¼ teaspoon salt (optional) ⅛ teaspoon black pepper	½ cup pitted Kalamata olives, chopped ¼ cup sun-dried tomatoes, thinly sliced 1½ cups hot water Hummus

1. Preheat a waffle iron. 2. In a large bowl, combine flour, rosemary, baking powder, salt (if desired), and pepper. Stir in olives and sun-dried tomatoes, then whisk in hot water until the batter is thick but thoroughly combined. 3. Spread about ½ to ¾ cup of batter onto the preheated waffle iron and cook according to the waffle iron's directions, for about 6 minutes. 4. Top the waffles with hummus and serve. Enjoy your savory Olive-Chickpea Waffles!

Per Serving: (1 waffle)

calories: 175 | fat: 5g | protein: 8g | carbs: 24g | fiber: 5g

Carrot Cake Date Balls

Prep time: 10 minutes | Cook time: 0 minutes | Makes 24 balls

1 cup shredded carrots 1 cup pitted dates ½ cup walnut pieces ¼ cup rolled oats 1 tablespoon coconut flakes	½ teaspoon ground cinnamon ¼ teaspoon ground ginger ⅛ teaspoon ground cloves ⅛ teaspoon ground nutmeg

1. Line a plate with parchment paper. 2. In a food processor, combine carrots, dates, walnuts, oats, coconut flakes, ginger, cloves, and nutmeg. Process until a paste forms. 3. Use a 1-tablespoon scoop to form the paste into balls. 4. Place the balls in a single layer on the prepared plate. Serve immediately or refrigerate in an airtight container for up to 5 days. Enjoy your Carrot Cake Date Balls!

Per Serving:

calories: 43 | fat: 2g | protein: 1g | carbs: 7g | fiber: 1g

Slow Cooker Versatile Seitan Balls

Prep time: 15 minutes | Cook time: 6 hours | Makes 34 balls

1½ cups vital wheat gluten	¼ teaspoon ground ginger
½ cup chickpea flour	¼ teaspoon ground cloves
1 tablespoon mushroom powder	¼ teaspoon ground sage
½ teaspoon dried oregano	½ teaspoon salt (optional)
½ teaspoon onion powder	½ cup tomato sauce, divided
¼ teaspoon garlic powder	1 teaspoon liquid smoke
¼ teaspoon nutmeg	1½ cups vegetable broth, divided

1. Mix the gluten, flour, mushroom powder, oregano, onion and garlic powders, nutmeg, ginger, cloves, sage, and salt (if desired) in a large bowl. 2. In a small bowl, add ¼ cup tomato sauce, ¼ cup water, liquid smoke, and ½ cup vegetable broth. Mix well. 3. Make a well in the center of the dry ingredients and pour in the tomato sauce mixture. Mix well and start to knead. Knead for 1 minute or until the dough becomes mildly elastic. You will see the dough slightly pull back as you are kneading and it will be a bit sticky. Pour remaining ¼ cup tomato sauce, 1 cup vegetable broth, and 3 cups water into the slow cooker. Stir. 4. Tear off small chunks of the dough, squeeze into a round shape, and drop into the liquid in the slow cooker. There will be forty-four balls. You can also make seventeen larger balls and cut them after cooking and cooling. Or make two logs and cut into desired shapes. Cover and cook on low for 4 to 6 hours. They will grow in size as they cook. Check at 4 hours and see if you like the texture. They will become firmer as they sit in the refrigerator. 5. Remove from the pot and let cool. Store in the refrigerator for up to 5 days or freeze for up to 4 months.

Per Serving: (½ cup)

calories: 161 | fat: 1g | protein: 30g | carbs: 10g | fiber: 2g

Calorie Bomb Cookies

Prep time: 15 minutes | Cook time: 30 minutes | Makes 24 cookies

4 cups old-fashioned rolled oats	water
1½ cups whole wheat flour	2 tablespoons chia seeds or ground flaxseeds
1 teaspoon baking powder	2 teaspoons vanilla extract
½ teaspoon salt (optional)	1 cup dark chocolate chips
3 ripe bananas	1 cup raw walnut pieces
1 cup coconut sugar (optional)	½ cup raw sunflower seeds
⅓ cup coconut oil (optional)	½ cup unsweetened shredded coconut (optional)
¼ cup plus 2 tablespoons	

1. Preheat the oven to 350ºF (180ºC). Line two baking sheets with parchment paper. 2. Place 2 cups of the oats in a food processor or blender and pulse until they are finely ground. Transfer to a large bowl and add the flour, baking powder, salt (if desired), and remaining oats. 3. Combine the bananas, sugar, oil (if desired), water, chia seeds, and vanilla in the blender or food processor. Add to the oat mixture and stir with a sturdy wooden spoon until combined. Add the chocolate chips, walnuts, sunflower seeds, and coconut. 4. With wet hands, form about ¼ cup dough. Flatten them to ¾ to 1 inch thick. 5. Bake for 30 minutes, or until golden brown. Allow to cool completely before removing from the baking sheets. Store in an airtight container for up to 1 week or freeze for up to 3 months. Wrap in parchment paper for on-the-go eating.

Per Serving: (2 cookies)

calories: 491 | fat: 24g | protein: 9g | carbs: 68g | fiber: 9g

Guacamole

Prep time: 10 minutes | Cook time: 0 minutes | Makes 2 cups

3 to 4 small avocados or 2 large avocados, diced	¾ teaspoon ground cumin
½ tablespoon lemon or lime juice	2 tablespoons chopped cilantro
¼ cup finely diced red, white, or yellow onion	½ medium tomato, chopped
1 teaspoon minced garlic	Pinch of salt (optional)
	Freshly ground pepper, to taste

1. In a medium bowl, mash the avocados with a fork to the desired consistency. 2. Add the lemon (or lime) juice, onion, garlic, cumin, cilantro, tomato, salt (if desired), and pepper, and mix well.

Per Serving:

calories: 249 | fat: 22g | protein: 4g | carbs: 15g | fiber: 10g

Garlic Hummus

Prep time: 10 minutes | Cook time: 0 minutes | Makes 3 cups

3 garlic cloves	Juice of 2 lemons
2 (15-ounce / 425-g) cans chickpeas, drained and rinsed	¼ cup tahini
	½ teaspoon salt
3 tablespoons extra-virgin olive oil, plus more as needed (optional)	½ teaspoon ground cumin
	1 tablespoon sesame seeds, for garnish (optional)

1. In a blender, combine the garlic, chickpeas, olive oil, lemon juice, tahini, salt, and cumin and blend until smooth and creamy. Add a bit more oil or water if you prefer a thinner consistency. To serve, spoon it into a bowl, drizzle with a little more olive oil, and garnish with sesame seeds (if using).

Per Serving:

calories: 58 | fat: 4g | protein: 2g | carbs: 5g | fiber: 2g

Gluten-Free Energy Crackers

Prep time: 25 minutes | Cook time: 40 minutes | Serves 6

¼ cup flax seeds	¼ cup peanuts, crushed
¼ cup chia seeds	¼ cup cashews, crushed
¾ cup water	¼ cup sesame seeds
1 tablespoon garlic, minced	¼ teaspoon paprika powder
½ tablespoon onion flakes	Salt and pepper to taste
½ cup pumpkin seeds, chopped	(optional)

1. Preheat the oven to 350ºF (180ºC). 2. Take a large bowl and combine the water, garlic, onion flakes, and paprika. Whisk until everything is combined thoroughly. Add the flax seeds, chia seeds, pumpkin seeds, peanuts, cashews, and sesame seeds to the bowl. Stir everything well, while adding pinches of salt (if desired) and pepper to taste, until it is thoroughly combined. 3. Line a baking sheet with parchment paper and spread out the mixture in a thin and even layer across the parchment paper. Bake for 20 to 25 minutes. Remove the pan from the oven and flip over the flat chunk so that the other side can crisp. Cut the chunk into squares or triangles, depending on preference and put the pan back into the oven and bake until the bars have turned golden brown, around 30 minutes. 4. Allow the crackers to cool before serving or storing.

Per Serving:

calories: 209 | fat: 16g | protein: 7g | carbs: 10g | fiber: 6g

Creamy Roasted Red Pepper Hummus

Prep time: 20 minutes | Cook time: 0 minutes | Serves 8

1 (15-ounce /425-g) can chickpeas, 3 tablespoons aquafaba (chickpea liquid from the can) reserved, remaining liquid drained, rinsed	1 teaspoon Hungarian paprika
	½ teaspoon ground cumin
	¼ teaspoon freshly ground black pepper
¼ cup tahini	2 garlic cloves, peeled and stemmed
1 tablespoon freshly squeezed lemon juice	2 roasted red peppers

1. Pour the chickpeas into a bowl and fill the bowl with water. Gently rub the chickpeas between your hands until you feel the skins coming off. Add more water to the bowl and let the skins float to the surface. Using your hand, scoop out the skins. Drain some of the water and repeat this step once more to remove as many of the chickpea skins as possible. Drain to remove all the water. Set the chickpeas aside. 2. In a food processor or high-speed blender, combine the reserved aquafaba, tahini, and lemon juice. Process for 2 minutes. 3. Add the paprika, cumin, black pepper, garlic, and red peppers. Purée until the red peppers are incorporated. 4. Add the chickpeas and blend for 2 to 3 minutes, or until the hummus is smooth. 5. Refrigerate leftovers in an airtight container for up to 1 week.

Per Serving:

calories: 99 | fat: 5g | protein: 4g | carbs: 11g | fiber: 3g

Toasted Protein Mushroom Rolls

Prep time: 20 minutes | Cook time: 15 minutes | Serves 6

¼ cup raw cashews, soaked for 1 hour	4 ounces (113 g) button mushrooms
1 tablespoon plus 2 teaspoons dairy-free milk	¼ cup dairy-free butter, divided
1 teaspoon lemon juice	2 tablespoons raw shelled hempseed
¼ teaspoon salt (optional)	9 slices whole-grain bread
Pinch of ground black pepper	

1. Add cashews, milk, lemon juice, salt (if desired), and pepper to a food processor. Process until smooth. 2. Clean mushrooms and finely chop. 3. Heat 1 tablespoon butter over medium-high heat in a small skillet. Add chopped mushrooms and sauté for 5 minutes. Turn off the heat and add the cashew mixture and hempseed. Stir well. 4. Preheat the oven to 425ºF (220ºC). 5. Cut crusts off of the bread and leave in a square shape. Roll each square thin with a rolling pin. You will be rolling up these squares. Spread 1 tablespoon mushroom mixture onto each square and roll up. 6. Melt remaining butter. 7. Cut rolls in half and roll in melted butter. Place rolls on cookie sheets and bake for 8 minutes or until browned.

Per Serving: (3 rolls)

calories: 261 | fat: 15g | protein: 18g | carbs: 25g | fiber: 4g

Cacao Crush Smoothie

Prep time: 5 minutes | Cook time: 0 minutes | Serves 1

1½ cups unsweetened almond milk	½ teaspoon ground cinnamon
½ cup frozen cauliflower	½ teaspoon pure vanilla extract
¼ avocado, peeled	
1 tablespoon cacao powder	

1. In a high-powered blender, combine the almond milk, cauliflower, avocado, cacao powder, cinnamon, and vanilla until smooth and creamy. 2. Serve immediately over a glass of ice.

Per Serving:

calories: 254 | fat: 7g | protein: 15g | carbs: 32g | fiber: 6g

Basic Oil-Free Hummus

Prep time: 10 minutes | Cook time: 0 minutes | Makes 1½ cups

1 (15-ounce / 425-g) can chickpeas, drained and rinsed
1 tablespoon tahini
¼ teaspoon garlic powder
¼ teaspoon ground cumin
¼ cup lemon juice
1/16 teaspoon cayenne
¼ teaspoon za'atar

1. In a food processor, combine the chickpeas, tahini, garlic powder, cumin, lemon juice, cayenne, and za'atar. Process until smooth and creamy.

Per Serving:

calories: 136 | fat: 6g | protein: 3g | carbs: 21g | fiber: 3g

Mixed Bag Chocolate walnut Protein Bars

Prep time: 20 minutes | Cook time: 35 minutes | Serves 8

3 tablespoons peanut butter
3 tablespoons maple syrup (optional)
1½ tablespoons coconut oil (optional)
1 tablespoon ground chia seeds
1¼ cups quick-cooking oats
½ cup walnuts
½ cup dairy-free chocolate
chips
⅓ cup coconut sugar (optional)
¼ cup raw shelled hempseed
3 tablespoons protein powder
½ teaspoon ground cinnamon
¼ teaspoon salt (optional)

1. Preheat the oven to 350ºF (180ºC). 2. Prepare an 8-inch square baking dish with parchment paper coming up on the sides on two opposite ends. Not over the top, just the sides. This makes for easier removal. 3. Add the peanut butter, maple syrup, and coconut oil (if desired) to a small saucepan. Heat to melt the peanut butter and stir well. Take off heat and let cool a bit. 4. Mix the ground chia seeds and 3 tablespoons water in a small bowl and set aside. 5. Add the oats, walnuts, chocolate chips, sugar, hempseed, protein powder, cinnamon, and salt (if desired) to a large bowl. Mix well. Add the chia mixture and peanut butter mixture to the bowl of dry ingredients and mix well. 6. Pour the mixture into the prepared dish and press down with your fingers to make the mix firm and pressed into all corners. 7. Bake for 30 to 35 minutes. The bars will get harder as they cool, so don't overbake. 8. Let cool on a wire rack. To remove, grab hold of the extra parchment paper on the opposite ends of the dish and lift. Place on a cutting board and slice into bars that are about 2 inches wide and then in half at 4 inches long.

Per Serving:

calories: 172 | fat: 9g | protein: 9g | carbs: 17g | fiber: 2g

Classic Italian Mushrooms

Prep time: 10 minutes | Cook time: 2 hours | Serves 4 to 6

2 pounds (907 g) white button mushrooms, stemmed
4 garlic cloves, minced
1 medium onion, sliced into half-moons
3 to 5 tablespoons store-
bought low-sodium vegetable broth
3 teaspoons Italian seasoning
Ground black pepper
Salt (optional)

1. Cut any extra-large mushrooms in half. Place the mushrooms in the slow cooker. Add the garlic and onion. 2. Pour in the broth and sprinkle with the Italian seasoning. Season with black pepper and salt (if using). Stir to combine. Cover and cook on Low for 2 hours, or until the mushrooms are cooked through.

Per Serving:

calories: 68 | fat: 1g | protein: 8g | carbs: 12g | fiber: 3g

Sweet Potato and Black Bean Quesadillas

Prep time: 10 minutes | Cook time: 20 minutes | Serves 4 to 6

Black Bean Spread:
1 (15-ounce / 425-g) can black beans, drained and rinsed
2 to 4 tablespoons chopped fresh cilantro stems and leaves
1 scallion, green and white parts, thinly sliced
1 tablespoon lime juice
1 teaspoon chipotle hot
sauce
¼ teaspoon red miso paste
⅛ teaspoon garlic powder
Quesadillas:
1 pound (454 g) sweet potatoes, peeled and shredded
4 to 6 (8-inch) whole-grain tortillas
Hot sauce, for serving

Make the Black Bean Spread: 1. In a small bowl, using a fork, mash the beans to a creamy texture. 2. Mix in the cilantro, scallion, lime juice, hot sauce, miso, and garlic powder. Make the Quesadillas: 3. Heat a large nonstick skillet over medium heat. 4. Put the sweet potatoes in the skillet, and cook, stirring every few minutes, for about 10 minutes, or until tender and browned. Transfer to a plate. 5. Wipe out the skillet, and return to the stove. 6. Divide the bean spread (about ¼ cup to 6 tablespoons per tortilla) among the tortillas, and spread evenly. 7. Divide the sweet potatoes (about ¼ cup per tortilla) onto half of each tortilla, fold in half, and press gently. 8. Place the tortillas in the hot skillet, and cook for 2 to 5 minutes per side, or until the tortillas are golden brown. Remove from the heat. 9. Serve the quesadillas with hot sauce.

Per Serving:

calories: 201 | fat: 1g | protein: 6g | carbs: 7g | fiber: 41g

Pepita and Almond Squares

Prep time: 20 minutes | Cook time: 15 minutes | Makes 16 squares

1 cup almonds, coarsely chopped	coconut
1 cup old-fashioned oats	¼ cup raw shelled hempseed
⅔ cup pepitas	⅓ cup peanut butter
⅔ cup dried cranberries	⅔ cup brown rice syrup
½ cup unsweetened shredded	¼ cup maple syrup (optional)
	2 teaspoons vanilla extract

1. Line an 8-inch square baking dish with parchment paper and come up about 3 inches on opposite sides. This will act as a handle to remove the squares from the dish. 2. In a large mixing bowl, add the almonds, oats, pepitas, cranberries, coconut, and hempseed. Mix well. Stir in the peanut butter and try to get it evenly combined. You can use your fingers when most of it is worked in. 3. Add the brown rice syrup, maple syrup (if desired), and vanilla to a small saucepan. Bring to a boil and continue boiling until it reaches the hard ball stage, 260°F (127°C), on a candy thermometer. When this temperature is reached, quickly pour over the almond mixture and stir well. It will start to harden up quickly. Pour into the prepared dish and press down firmly into the dish and as evenly as possible. Refrigerate for at least 30 minutes. 4. Grab the "handles" of the parchment paper and lift out of the dish. Place on a cutting sheet and slice into sixteen squares.

Per Serving: (2 squares)

calories: 198 | fat: 11g | protein: 12g | carbs: 22g | fiber: 4g

Pressure Cooker Tender Patties

Prep time: 10 minutes | Cook time: 5 minutes | Makes 2 cups

¾ cup vital wheat gluten	¼ teaspoon onion powder
¼ cup chickpea flour	¼ teaspoon paprika
2 tablespoons nutritional yeast	2¼ cups vegetable broth, divided
½ teaspoon dried basil	1 teaspoon extra virgin olive oil (optional)
½ teaspoon salt (optional)	½ teaspoon tamari
½ teaspoon poultry seasoning	2 tablespoons tomato sauce
¼ teaspoon garlic powder	

1. Add the gluten, flour, nutritional yeast, basil, salt (if desired), poultry seasoning, garlic and onion powders, and paprika to a large bowl. 2. Mix ¾ cup vegetable broth, oil (if desired), and tamari in a small bowl. Pour the wet mixture into the dry ingredients. 3. Mix and then knead for about 2 to 3 minutes or until elastic. It should be stretchy and pull back but still pliable. Divide the dough into eight pieces. Use your fingers to squeeze and work around into a patty measuring about 3 to 4 inches in diameter. 4. Place in an electric pressure cooker. 5. Add 1½ cups water, 1½ cups vegetable broth, and the tomato sauce to a small bowl, stir, and then pour over the seitan cutlets in the pressure cooker. Close the lid, making sure the top knob is turned to sealing. Press Manual on the front of the pot. Push button to 4 (meaning 4 minutes). In a few seconds, the pressure cooker will make a click and start to build pressure. It will take about 15 minutes to build pressure and cook. Leave the cutlets in the pot to set. They will cook more as the pressure is naturally releasing. Don't vent. 6. After about an hour, go ahead and vent. It may already have cooled completely, but vent to make sure all of the pressure has been released and then open the lid. 7. Remove the cutlets from the liquid and set aside to cool. You can eat them right away, add to a recipe, or keep in the fridge overnight. They are great the next day and keep well in the freezer.

Per Serving: (½ cup)

calories: 247 | fat: 2g | protein: 30g | carbs: 16g | fiber: 3g

Pineapple, Peach, and Mango Salsa

Prep time: 15 minutes | Cook time: 2 to 3 hours | Makes about 6 cups

1 medium onion, finely diced	1 (15 ounces / 425 g) can no-sugar-added sliced peaches in juice, drained and finely diced
2 garlic cloves, minced	
1 medium orange, red, or yellow bell pepper, finely diced	½ teaspoon ground cumin
	1 teaspoon paprika
1 (20 ounces / 567 g) can crushed pineapple in juice	Juice of 1 lime
1 (15 ounces / 425 g) can no-sugar-added mango in juice, drained and finely diced	3 to 4 tablespoons chopped fresh mint (about 10 to 15 leaves)

1. Put the onion, garlic, and bell pepper in the slow cooker. Add the pineapple and its juices, the mango, and the peaches. Sprinkle the cumin and paprika into the slow cooker. Add the lime juice and stir well to combine. 2. Cover and cook on Low for 2 to 3 hours, or until the onion and peppers are cooked through and softened. Let the salsa cool slightly, then stir in the mint just before serving.

Per Serving:

calories: 36 | fat: 0g | protein: 1g | carbs: 9g | fiber: 1g

Chapter 7 Vegetables and Sides

Summer Squash and Blossom Sauté with Mint and Peas

Prep time: 10 minutes | Cook time: 10 minutes | Serves 4

½ cup fresh or frozen peas 1 pound (454 g) mixed zucchini and pattypan squash 1 tablespoon extra-virgin coconut oil (optional)	15 large zucchini blossoms, stems removed and chopped into ½-inch pieces A handful of fresh mint leaves, torn

1. If using fresh peas, boil them in a saucepan of water for about 3 minutes until tender, then drain and set aside. 2. Slice the zucchini into ½-inch pieces and cut pattypan squash into ½-inch wedges. Heat oil in a wide skillet over medium-high heat, and sauté the squash, stirring frequently, until tender and slightly browned, about 2 to 3 minutes. Add the peas and zucchini blossoms, cook for another minute until the blossoms are softened and the peas are heated through. Remove from heat and serve immediately. For any leftovers, store in the refrigerator for up to a day or two. Enjoy your Summer Squash and Blossom Sauté with Mint and Peas!

Per Serving:

calories: 262 | fat: 8g | protein: 17g | carbs: 42g | fiber: 14g

Spicy Carrots with Coriander

Prep time: 15 minutes | Cook time: 0 minutes | Serves 2

3 cups shredded carrots 4 garlic cloves, minced ¼ cup rice vinegar 1 tablespoon maple syrup (optional) 1 tablespoon ground coriander 1 teaspoon red pepper flakes	½ teaspoon freshly ground black pepper ¼ tablespoon cayenne pepper 1 teaspoon dried dill (optional) 1 teaspoon dried parsley (optional)

1. In a large mixing bowl, mix together the carrots, garlic, rice vinegar, and maple syrup (if using). Add the red pepper flakes, coriander, cayenne pepper, and black pepper, and stir well to coat the carrots with the spicy seasoning. 2. For added flavor, you can also include dried dill and parsley. Let the mixture sit for at least 10 minutes to allow the flavors to meld, then enjoy your spicy and delicious carrots with a kick of coriander!

Per Serving:

calories: 101 | fat: 0g | protein: 2g | carbs: 23g | fiber: 4g

Chili-Lime Corn

Prep time: 10 minutes | Cook time: 3 hours | Serves 4 to 6

4½ cups frozen corn 1 small red onion, diced 1 small green bell pepper, diced Juice and zest of 2 limes	2 teaspoons chili powder 1 teaspoon ground cumin 1 teaspoon garlic powder Salt (optional)

1. In a slow cooker, combine corn, onion, bell pepper, lime juice and zest, chili powder, cumin, garlic powder, and salt (if using). Mix well. 2. Cover and cook on Low for 3 hours. Store any leftovers in an airtight container in the refrigerator for 3 to 4 days or freeze for up to 1 month. Reheat in the microwave when ready to enjoy again. Enjoy the delicious chili-lime flavor!

Per Serving:

calories: 188 | fat: 2g | protein: 7g | carbs: 44g | fiber: 7g

Grilled Eggplant "Steaks"

Prep time: 10 minutes | Cook time: 10 minutes | Serves 4

3 tablespoons balsamic vinegar Juice of 1 lemon 2 tablespoons low-sodium soy sauce	Freshly ground black pepper, to taste 1 large eggplant, stemmed and cut into ¾-inch slices

1. Prepare the grill. 2. Combine the balsamic vinegar, lemon juice, soy sauce, and pepper in a small bowl. 3. Brush both sides of the eggplant slices with the marinade. 4. Place the eggplant on the hot grill and cook on each side for 4 to 5 minutes, brushing periodically with additional marinade.

Per Serving:

calories: 51 | fat: 0g | protein: 2g | carbs: 11g | fiber: 4g

Ratatouille

Prep time: 30 minutes | Cook time: 25 minutes | Serves 4

1 medium red onion, peeled and diced	1 small zucchini, diced
1 medium red bell pepper, seeded and diced	4 cloves garlic, peeled and minced
1 medium eggplant, about 1 pound / 454 g, stemmed and diced	½ cup chopped basil
	1 large tomato, diced
	Salt and freshly ground black pepper, to taste

1. In a medium saucepan, sauté the onion over medium heat for 10 minutes. Add water as needed to prevent sticking. Stir in red pepper, eggplant, zucchini, and garlic. Cook, covered, for 15 minutes, stirring occasionally. 2. Stir in basil and tomatoes, and season with salt and pepper.

Per Serving:

calories: 34 | fat: 0g | protein: 1g | carbs: 7g | fiber: 2g

Fluffy Mashed Potatoes with Gravy

Prep time: 10 minutes | Cook time: 15 minutes | Serves 6

Mashed Potatoes:	divided
8 red or Yukon Gold potatoes, cut into 1-inch cubes	¼ cup gluten-free or whole-wheat flour
½ cup plant-based milk (here or here)	½ teaspoon garlic powder
1 teaspoon garlic powder	½ teaspoon onion powder
1 teaspoon onion powder	¼ teaspoon freshly ground black pepper
Gravy:	¼ teaspoon dried thyme
2 cups vegetable broth,	¼ teaspoon dried sage

1. In a large stockpot, bring water to a boil over high heat. Carefully add the potatoes and boil for 15 minutes or until fork-tender. Drain the liquid and return the potatoes to the pot. Mash them until smooth, then stir in milk, garlic powder, and onion powder. 2. For the gravy, whisk together ½ cup of broth and flour in a medium saucepan until no dry flour remains. Gradually whisk in the remaining 1½ cups of broth. Stir in garlic powder, onion powder, pepper, thyme, and sage. Bring the gravy to a boil, then reduce the heat to low and simmer for 10 minutes, stirring occasionally. Serve the gravy with the mashed potatoes.

Per Serving:

calories: 260 | fat: 1g | protein: 8g | carbs: 56g | fiber: 4g

Tangy Cabbage, Apples, and Potatoes

Prep time: 15 minutes | Cook time: 3 to 4 hours | Serves 4 to 6

6 red or yellow potatoes (about 2 pounds / 907 g), unpeeled and cut into 1½-inch chunks	sodium vegetable broth
	½ cup apple juice, apple cider, or hard apple cider
½ medium onion, diced	2 tablespoons apple cider vinegar
2 apples, peeled, cored, and diced	2 teaspoons ground mustard, or 1 tablespoon spicy brown mustard
½ teaspoon ground cinnamon	1 teaspoon fennel seeds
½ medium head green cabbage, sliced	1 bay leaf
1 cup store-bought low-	Ground black pepper
	Salt (optional)

1. In the slow cooker, layer the potatoes, onion, and apples. Sprinkle cinnamon over the apples and top with cabbage. 2. Whisk together broth, apple juice, vinegar, mustard, fennel, bay leaf, pepper, and salt (if using) in a small bowl. Pour the mixture over the cabbage. 3. Cover and cook on High for 3 to 4 hours or on Low for 6 to 8 hours. Remove and discard the bay leaf before serving.

Per Serving:

calories: 266 | fat: 1g | protein: 7g | carbs: 62g | fiber: 10g

Roasted Veggies with Tofu

Prep time: 10 minutes | Cook time: 30 minutes | Serves 4

1½ pounds (680 g) mixed vegetables	¼ cup vegetable broth
1 pound (454 g) extra-firm tofu or tempeh	2 tablespoons spice blend
	Salt and black pepper (optional)

1. Preheat your oven to 400ºF (205ºC) and line two baking sheets with parchment paper. 2. Chop the vegetables into equal-sized pieces and cube the tofu. 3. Divide the vegetables and tofu between the prepared baking sheets. Drizzle with the broth and evenly sprinkle the spices over the baking sheets. Toss everything well to ensure even coating and season with salt (if desired) and pepper. 4. Bake the trays uncovered for about 30 minutes or until the vegetables are cooked through and starting to brown. If needed, rotate the baking sheets halfway through to ensure even cooking. Once ready, serve and enjoy your delicious Roasted Veggies with Tofu!

Per Serving:

calories: 218 | fat: 7g | protein: 16g | carbs: 25g | fiber: 8g

Baked Spaghetti Squash with Spicy Lentil Sauce

Prep time: 15 minutes | Cook time: 55 minutes | Serves 4

2 small spaghetti squash (about 1 pound / 454 g each), halved	2 teaspoons crushed red pepper flakes, or to taste
Salt and freshly ground black pepper, to taste	¼ cup tomato paste
1 medium yellow onion, peeled and diced small	1 cup cooked green lentils
3 cloves garlic, peeled and minced	1 cup vegetable stock, or low-sodium vegetable broth, plus more as needed
	Chopped parsley

1. Preheat the oven to 350ºF (180ºC). 2. Season the cut sides of the squash with salt and pepper. Place the squash halves, cut side down, on a baking sheet, and bake for 45 to 55 minutes until tender. 3. While the squash bakes, sauté the onion in a large saucepan for 5 minutes. Add water as needed to prevent sticking. Stir in garlic, crushed red pepper flakes, tomato paste, and ½ cup of water. Cook for 5 minutes. Add the lentils and heat through. Season with salt. Purée the lentil mixture using an immersion blender or regular blender until smooth, adding vegetable stock as needed to create a creamy sauce. 4. To serve, scoop the spaghetti squash flesh onto plates, top with lentil sauce, and garnish with parsley. Enjoy!

Per Serving:

calories: 94 | fat: 0g | protein: 6g | carbs: 18g | fiber: 5g

Loaded Frijoles

Prep time: 10 minutes | Cook time: 20 minutes | Serves 6

1 tablespoon avocado oil (optional)	1 teaspoon ground cumin
1 yellow onion, finely chopped	2 (15-ounce / 425-g) cans pinto beans, undrained
3 garlic cloves, minced	¼ cup tomato sauce
2 teaspoons chili powder	Sea salt, to taste (optional)

1. In a 4-quart pan, heat avocado oil (if using) over medium-high heat. Sauté the onion for 5 minutes. 2. Add garlic and cook for 30 seconds, then add chili powder and cumin, cooking for another 30 seconds. 3. Stir in the beans and tomato sauce. Taste and add salt (if using), if needed. 4. Mash the beans or use an immersion blender to achieve the desired consistency. Cook over medium-low heat for 15 minutes, or until the beans thicken. Add water if the beans become too thick. 5. Store the Frijoles in an airtight container in the fridge for up to 1 week or in the freezer for several months. Enjoy!

Per Serving:

calories: 142 | fat: 3g | protein: 7g | carbs: 22g | fiber: 6g

Blackened Sprouts

Prep time: 10 minutes | Cook time: 20 minutes | Serves 4

1 pound (454 g) fresh Brussels sprouts, trimmed and halved	Sea salt and ground black pepper, to taste
2 tablespoons avocado oil (optional)	1 cup walnut halves
	1 tablespoon pure maple syrup (optional)

1. Preheat your oven to 425ºF (220ºC) and line a baking sheet with parchment paper or grease it well. 2. In a medium bowl, toss the sprouts with oil (if using) and season with salt and pepper to taste. Arrange them in a single layer on the prepared baking sheet. 3. Roast the sprouts for about 20 minutes or until the edges start to blacken, giving them a delicious charred flavor. 4. While the sprouts are roasting, place the walnuts in a bowl and drizzle with maple syrup (if using). Toss until the walnuts are well coated. In the last 3 minutes of roasting time, place the coated walnuts on the same baking sheet as the sprouts to toast and caramelize. 5. Once done, let the blackened sprouts and caramelized walnuts cool slightly before serving. Enjoy this flavorful and nutritious dish!

Per Serving:

calories: 254 | fat: 20g | protein: 6g | carbs: 16g | fiber: 5g

Fermented Carrots with Turmeric and Ginger

Prep time: 15 minutes | Cook time: 0 minutes | Makes 8 cups

10 medium-large carrots, grated	grated
½ medium cabbage, cored and thinly sliced with 1 leaf reserved	1 (2-inch) piece fresh ginger, peeled and finely grated
1 (3-inch) piece fresh turmeric, peeled and finely	1 small shallot, finely chopped
	5 teaspoons fine sea salt (optional)

1. Combine carrots, cabbage, turmeric, ginger, shallot, and salt (if using) in a large bowl. Mix well until vegetables are juicy and wilted. Pack the mixture into a wide-mouthed jar or fermentation crock, ensuring it's submerged in liquid. Add a weight to keep the vegetables submerged, cover, and ferment for 10 days in a cool, dark place. 2. After 10 days, taste the carrots. If the desired tanginess and flavor are achieved, transfer to the fridge. Otherwise, reseal and ferment for a few more days, checking the taste. The fermented carrots will keep for months in the fridge, and their flavor will continue to develop gradually.

Per Serving: (1 cup)

calories: 37 | fat: 0g | protein: 1g | carbs: 9g | fiber: 3g

Indian Spiced Eggplant

Prep time: 20 minutes | Cook time: 25 minutes | Serves 4

2 medium onions, peeled and diced	2 teaspoons cumin seeds, toasted and ground
1 large red bell pepper, seeded and diced	1 teaspoon coriander seeds, toasted and ground
2 medium eggplants, stemmed, peeled, and cut into ½-inch dice	½ teaspoon crushed red pepper flakes
2 large tomatoes, finely chopped	Pinch cloves
	Salt, to taste (optional)
3 tablespoons grated ginger	½ bunch cilantro, leaves and tender stems, finely chopped

1. Sauté onions and red pepper in a large saucepan over medium heat for 10 minutes. Add water as needed to prevent sticking. 2. Add eggplant, tomatoes, ginger, cumin, coriander, crushed red pepper flakes, and cloves. Cook until eggplant is tender, about 15 minutes. Season with salt (optional) and garnish with cilantro before serving. Enjoy your flavorful and aromatic Indian Spiced Eggplant!

Per Serving:
calories: 111 | fat: 1g | protein: 4g | carbs: 25g | fiber: 9g

Glowing, Fermented Vegetable Tangle

Prep time: 15 minutes | Cook time: 0 minutes |Makes 2 quarts

1 fennel bulb, cored	ginger, peeled and finely grated
1 head green cabbage, quartered cored and save the flexible outer leaves	1 (2-inch) piece of fresh turmeric root, peeled and finely grated or 2 teaspoons turmeric powder
6 medium carrots, shredded	
2 medium beets, shredded	2 teaspoons cumin seeds
2 apples, peeled, cored and shredded	2 teaspoons chili flakes
1 (2-inch) piece of fresh	Sea salt, to taste (optional)

1. Shave fennel and cabbage thinly with a mandoline over a large bowl. 2. Add carrots, beets, apples, ginger, turmeric, cumin seeds, and chili flakes. Season with sea salt and massage the vegetables for 5 minutes to release liquid. 3. Pack the mixture into jars, leaving 1 inch of space at the top. Place a cabbage leaf on top, secure the lid, and put the jars in plastic bags to prevent staining. Store in a cool place for 3 weeks, checking for desired taste and texture. Once ready, remove cabbage leaf toppers and refrigerate. Enjoy your tangy and flavorful fermented vegetables!

Per Serving: (½ quart)
calories: 187 | fat: 1g | protein: 6g | carbs: 44g | fiber: 14g

Sautéed Collard Greens

Prep time: 10 minutes | Cook time: 25 minutes | Serves 4

1½ pounds (680 g) collard greens	½ teaspoon onion powder
1 cup vegetable broth	⅛ teaspoon freshly ground black pepper
½ teaspoon garlic powder	

1. Remove the hard middle stems from the greens, then roughly chop the leaves into 2-inch pieces. 2. In a large saucepan, mix together the vegetable broth, garlic powder, onion powder, and pepper. Bring to a boil over medium-high heat, then add the chopped greens. Reduce the heat to low, and cover. 3. Cook for 20 minutes, stirring well every 4 to 5 minutes, and serve. (If you notice that the liquid has completely evaporated and the greens are beginning to stick to the bottom of the pan, stir in a few extra tablespoons of vegetable broth or water.)

Per Serving:
calories: 28 | fat: 1g | protein: 3g | carbs: 4g | fiber: 2g

Stir-Fried Vegetables with Miso and Sake

Prep time: 25 minutes | Cook time: 10 minutes | Serves 4

¼ cup mellow white miso	strips
½ cup vegetable stock, or low-sodium vegetable broth	1 large head broccoli, cut into florets
¼ cup sake	½ pound (227 g) snow peas, trimmed
1 medium yellow onion, peeled and thinly sliced	2 cloves garlic, peeled and minced
1 large carrot, peeled, cut in half lengthwise, and then cut into half-moons on the diagonal	½ cup chopped cilantro (optional)
1 medium red bell pepper, seeded and cut into ½-inch	Salt and freshly ground black pepper, to taste

1. Whisk together the miso, vegetable stock, and sake in a small bowl and set aside. 2. Heat a large skillet over high heat. Add the onion, carrot, red pepper, and broccoli and stir-fry for 4 to 5 minutes. Add water 1 to 2 tablespoons at a time to keep the vegetables from sticking to the pan. Add the snow peas and stir-fry for another 4 minutes. Add the garlic and cook for 30 seconds. Add the miso mixture and cook until heated through. 3. Remove the pan from the heat and add the cilantro (if using). Season with salt and pepper.

Per Serving:
calories: 135 | fat: 1g | protein: 7g | carbs: 24g | fiber: 7g

Savory Slow Cooker Stuffing

Prep time: 20 minutes | Cook time: 4 hours 45 minutes | Serves 5 to 7

Nonstick cooking spray (optional)	white button mushrooms, diced
2 (12 ounces / 340 g) packages stuffing cubes (about 12 cups)	2 teaspoons dried sage
	1 teaspoon poultry seasoning
2 tablespoons ground flaxseed	1 teaspoon marjoram
5 tablespoons water	1 teaspoon crushed or ground fennel seed
2 small or 1 large onion, diced (about 2 cups)	⅓ cup chopped fresh parsley
	Ground black pepper
6 large celery stalks, diced (about 2 cups)	Salt (optional)
1 (8 ounces / 227 g) package	3½ to 5 cups store-bought low-sodium vegetable broth, divided

1. Coat the inside of the slow cooker with cooking spray (if using) or line it with a slow cooker liner. Place the dry stuffing cubes in the slow cooker. In a small bowl, stir together the flaxseed and water to make 2 flax eggs. Set aside. 2. In a cast-iron or nonstick skillet over medium-high heat, dry sauté the onions, celery, and mushrooms for 5 to 7 minutes, or until the onions are translucent, adding a splash of water or broth to avoid sticking. Stir in the sage, poultry seasoning, marjoram, fennel seed, parsley, pepper, and salt (if using) and cook for another minute or so. Transfer the mixture to the slow cooker and add 3½ cups of broth, stirring to combine. Add more broth, ½ cup at a time, to achieve your desired consistency. 3. Cover and cook on High for 45 minutes, then turn the heat to Low and cook for 3 to 4 hours, until the stuffing reaches the consistency you prefer. Add more broth as needed during the cooking time for a moister stuffing.

Per Serving:

calories: 523 | fat: 7g | protein: 20g | carbs: 77g | fiber: 10g

Fennel and Green Cabbage Kraut

Prep time: 10 minutes | Cook time: 0 minutes | Makes 8 cups

1 medium green cabbage, cored and thinly sliced with 1 leaf reserved	mandoline or thinly sliced
	5 teaspoons fine sea salt (optional)
1 large fennel bulb, trimmed, cored, and shaved on a	2 teaspoons fennel seeds

1. Combine the cabbage, shaved or sliced fennel, salt, if using, and fennel seeds in a large bowl and use clean hands to mix the vegetables together, squeezing and softening them until they are juicy and wilted. Transfer a handful of the mixture to a large widemouthed jar or a fermentation crock and press it down with your fist. Repeat with the remaining mixture, a handful at a time, and then add any liquid left in the bowl. The liquid should completely cover the mixture; if it does not, keep pressing the mixture down until it does. You should have at least 3 inches of headspace above the vegetables. Clean the edges of the jar or crock of any stray pieces of vegetable. 2. Place the reserved cabbage leaf on top of the vegetables. Add a weight, such as a small glass jar filled with water, a flat glass plate or lid, or a fermentation weight, to keep the vegetables submerged, then seal the jar or crock. Label and date it and put it in a cool, dark place for 10 days. 3. After 10 days, carefully remove the lid, as it might pop off because of the gases that have built up, then remove the weight and cabbage leaf and use a clean fork to remove a little of the kraut to taste. If the level of tanginess and complexity of flavor are to your liking, transfer the jar or crock to the fridge, or transfer the kraut to smaller jars and refrigerate. If not, replace the leaf and the weight, tighten the lid, set aside for a few more days, and taste again. Usually 2 to 3 weeks of fermentation results in a good flavor. The kraut will keep in the fridge for months. The flavor will continue to develop, but at a much slower rate.

Per Serving: (1 cup)

calories: 39 | fat: 0g | protein: 2g | carbs: 9g | fiber: 4g

Aloo Gobi (Potato and Cauliflower Curry)

Prep time: 25 minutes | Cook time: 27 minutes | Serves 4

1 medium yellow onion, peeled and diced	into ½-inch dice
	1 teaspoon ground cumin
1 tablespoon grated ginger	1 teaspoon ground coriander
2 cloves garlic, peeled and minced	1 teaspoon crushed red pepper flakes
½ jalapeño pepper, seeded and minced	½ teaspoon turmeric
	¼ teaspoon ground cloves
2 medium tomatoes, diced	2 bay leaves
1 medium head cauliflower, cut into florets	1 cup green peas
	¼ cup chopped cilantro or mint
1 pound (454 g) Yukon Gold or other waxy potatoes, cut	

1. In a large saucepan, sauté the onion over medium heat for 7 to 8 minutes. Add water as needed to prevent sticking. Stir in ginger, garlic, and jalapeño pepper, and cook for an additional 3 minutes. Add tomatoes, cauliflower, potatoes, cumin, coriander, crushed red pepper flakes, turmeric, cloves, and bay leaves. Cover and cook for 10 to 12 minutes until the vegetables are tender. Stir in peas and cook for an additional 5 minutes. 2. Remove the bay leaves and garnish with cilantro or mint before serving.

Per Serving:

calories: 163 | fat: 0g | protein: 6g | carbs: 34g | fiber: 7g

Tangy Cabbage and Kale Slaw

Prep time: 10 minutes | Cook time: 0 minutes | Makes 3 cups

8 ounces (227 g) shredded cabbage	½ bunch kale, stemmed (if desired) and chopped small
½ bunch fresh cilantro, chopped	½ teaspoon salt (optional)
1 scallion, white and green parts, chopped	1 teaspoon extra-virgin olive oil (optional)
	Juice of 2 limes

1. In a large bowl, combine the cabbage, cilantro, scallion, kale, salt, olive oil (if using), and lime juice and mix well with your hands. Store in an airtight container for up to 3 days in the refrigerator.

Per Serving:

calories: 43 | fat: 1g | protein: 2g | carbs: 8g | fiber: 2g

Millet-Stuffed Portobello Mushrooms

Prep time: 20 minutes | Cook time: 1 hour 5 minutes | Serves 4

4 large portobello mushrooms, stemmed	⅔ cup millet
2 tablespoons low-sodium soy sauce	1 small yellow onion, peeled and diced small
3 cloves garlic, peeled and minced	1 medium red bell pepper, seeded and diced small
Freshly ground black pepper, to taste	1 fennel bulb, trimmed and diced
Filling:	3 cloves garlic, peeled and minced
2 cups low-sodium vegetable stock	2 sage leaves, minced
	Salt, to taste (optional)

1. Place the portobello mushrooms, stem side up, in a baking dish. 2. In a small bowl, combine soy sauce, minced garlic, and black pepper to make the marinade. Brush the marinade over each mushroom and set them aside. 3. In a medium saucepan, bring vegetable stock to a boil. Add millet and cook, covered, over medium heat for about 15 minutes or until tender. 4. Preheat the oven to 350ºF (180ºC). 5. In a large saucepan, sauté onion, red pepper, and fennel over medium heat for 10 minutes. Add water as needed to prevent sticking. Stir in minced garlic and sage leaves, then add cooked millet. Season with salt and pepper. Remove from heat. 6. Divide the millet mixture among the mushrooms, arranging them in the baking dish. Cover with foil and bake for 25 minutes. Remove the foil and bake for an additional 10 minutes.

Per Serving:

calories: 179 | fat: 1g | protein: 7g | carbs: 35g | fiber: 6g

Chickpea of the Sea Salad

Prep time: 15 minutes | Cook time: 4 hours | Serves 3 to 4

1 (1-pound / 454-g) bag dried chickpeas, rinsed and sorted to remove small stones and debris	1 tablespoon yellow mustard
	¼ cup diced dill pickles
	¼ cup finely diced onions
7 cups water	1 celery stalk, diced
¼ teaspoon baking soda	2 tablespoons rice vinegar
5 tablespoons plant-based mayonnaise	½ teaspoon kelp powder
	Ground black pepper
	Salt (optional)

1. In a slow cooker, combine the chickpeas, water, and baking soda. Cook on High for 4 hours or Low for 8 to 9 hours. Strain and discard the liquid. 2. Transfer 2 cups of the cooked chickpeas to a food processor and pulse 5 to 10 times to break them up without turning them into mush. Transfer the pulsed chickpeas to a medium bowl, reserving the remaining chickpeas for another recipe. 3. Add mayonnaise, mustard, pickles, onions, celery, vinegar, kelp powder, pepper, and salt (if using) to the bowl. Stir well to create the salad and chill before serving. Enjoy!

Per Serving:

calories: 313 | fat: 21g | protein: 8g | carbs: 25g | fiber: 7g

Braised Red Cabbage with Beans

Prep time: 25 minutes | Cook time: 38 minutes | Serves 4

1 large yellow onion, peeled and diced	cored and shredded
2 large carrots, peeled and diced	4 cups cooked navy beans, or 2 (15-ounce / 425-g) cans, drained and rinsed
2 celery stalks, diced	2 tart apples (such as Granny Smith), peeled, cored, and diced
2 teaspoons thyme	
1½ cups red wine	Salt and freshly ground black pepper, to taste
2 tablespoons Dijon mustard	
1 large head red cabbage,	

1. Place the onion, carrots, and celery in a large saucepan and sauté over medium heat for 7 to 8 minutes. Add water 1 to 2 tablespoons at a time to keep the vegetables from sticking to the pan. Add the thyme, red wine, and mustard and cook until the wine is reduced by half, about 10 minutes. 2. Add the cabbage, beans, and apples. Cook, covered, until the cabbage is tender, about 20 minutes. Season with salt and pepper.

Per Serving:

calories: 315 | fat: 1g | protein: 14g | carbs: 60g | fiber: 20g

Spring Steamed Vegetables with Savory Goji Berry Cream

Prep time: 15 minutes | Cook time: 10 minutes | Serves 6

Savory Goji Berry Cream:	(optional)
¼ cup dried goji berries	Salt and pepper, to taste
1 tablespoon apple cider vinegar	(optional)
1 tablespoon mellow or light miso	Vegetables:
1 tablespoon fresh lemon juice	1½ pounds (680 g) trimmed spring vegetables
1 (1-inch) piece of fresh ginger, peeled and chopped	Salt and pepper, to taste (optional)
1 teaspoon pure maple syrup (optional)	Garnishes:
3 tablespoons virgin olive oil	Scant ¼ cup walnut halves, toasted and chopped
	1 green onion, thinly sliced

1. Prepare the Savory Goji Berry Cream by soaking the goji berries and blending them with the listed ingredients until creamy. Set aside. 2. Trim the vegetables and steam them in a pot with 1 inch of water until tender. 3. Arrange the steamed vegetables on a serving platter and top with the Savory Goji Berry Cream. Garnish with chopped walnuts and sliced green onions. Enjoy your delicious and nutritious dish!

Per Serving:

calories: 136 | fat: 9g | protein: 5g | carbs: 17g | fiber: 5g

Lemony Steamed Kale with Olives

Prep time: 10 minutes | Cook time: 20 minutes | Serves 4

1 bunch kale, leaves chopped and stems minced	2 tablespoons vegetable broth
½ cup celery leaves, roughly chopped	¼ cup pitted Kalamata olives, chopped
½ bunch flat-leaf parsley, stems and leaves roughly chopped	Grated zest and juice of 1 lemon
4 garlic cloves, chopped	Salt and pepper (optional)

1. Prepare the kale by removing the tough stems and tearing the leaves into smaller pieces. Rinse the kale thoroughly under running water to remove any dirt or grit. 2. In a steamer basket set over a medium saucepan, place the kale, celery leaves, parsley, and minced garlic. Make sure the steamer basket fits securely over the saucepan. 3. Fill the saucepan with enough water so that it doesn't touch the bottom of the steamer basket. Cover the saucepan with a lid and bring the water to a boil over medium-high heat. Reduce the heat to medium and steam the kale mixture for about 15 minutes, or until it becomes tender and bright green. 4. Carefully remove the steamer basket from the saucepan and allow the excess moisture to drain. Gently squeeze the kale to remove any remaining water. Heat some vegetable or chicken broth in a large skillet over medium heat. Add the steamed kale mixture to the skillet and stir-fry it for about 5 minutes, or until it's heated through and well-coated with the broth. Remove the skillet from the heat and add pitted olives (such as Kalamata olives) along with freshly grated lemon zest and juice. Stir everything together to combine. Taste the dish and season with salt and pepper according to your preference. Keep in mind that olives can be quite salty, so you may not need much additional salt. Serve the Lemony Steamed Kale with Olives as a side dish or a light main course. It pairs well with grilled chicken or fish. Enjoy!

Per Serving:

calories: 41 | fat: 1g | protein: 2g | carbs: 7g | fiber: 2g

Vegetable Korma Curry

Prep time: 10 minutes | Cook time: 20 minutes | Serves 4

1 tablespoon extra-virgin olive oil (optional)	2 cups water, divided
2 garlic cloves, minced	1 cup softened cashews
2 tablespoons minced fresh ginger	1 tablespoon curry powder
½ small yellow onion, diced small	2 tablespoons tomato paste
1 medium sweet potato, peeled and cut into small cubes	½ cup frozen green beans
½ head cauliflower, cut into small florets (about 2 cups)	½ cup frozen peas
3 medium tomatoes, diced small	1 (15-ounce / 425-g) can light unsweetened coconut milk
Pinch of salt (optional)	2 cups cooked brown rice or quinoa, for serving
	Chopped fresh cilantro, for garnish
	Black pepper

1. In a large sauté pan, heat the oil over medium heat. Add the garlic, ginger, and onion and cook until browned and fragrant, about 5 minutes. Add the sweet potato, cauliflower, tomatoes, and salt (if using) and cook until the tomatoes begin to break down, about 5 minutes. Add 1 cup of water, stir until combined, and bring the mixture to a boil. Cook until the sweet potatoes are soft, about 10 minutes. 2. In a blender or food processor, combine the cashews with the remaining 1 cup water and blend until you have a smooth paste. 3. Add the blended cashews, curry powder, tomato paste, green beans, peas, and coconut milk to the pan and stir well to combine. Lower the heat to medium-low and simmer for 5 minutes. Taste and adjust the seasoning as desired. 4. Put ½ cup of rice into each serving bowl and top with the curry. Sprinkle with fresh cilantro and black pepper.

Per Serving:

calories: 535 | fat: 29g | protein: 14g | carbs: 55g | fiber: 8g

Shaved Fennel and Lemon Pickle

Prep time: 5 minutes | Cook time: 0 minutes | Serves 6

1 large fennel	more to taste
3 tablespoons freshly	¾ teaspoon fine sea salt, or
squeezed lemon juice, or	more to taste (optional)

1. Trim off the fennel stalks. Remove any tough outer layers from the fennel bulbs, quarter each one, and remove the cores. Shave on a mandoline or slice paper-thin with a sharp knife. Put the fennel in a medium bowl, add the lemon juice and salt, if using, and mix well to combine. Season to taste with more salt or lemon juice if necessary. Serve immediately, or store in a jar in the fridge for up to 1 week.

Per Serving:

calories: 14 | fat: 0g | protein: 1g | carbs: 3g | fiber: 1g

Gingered Brussels Sprout and Shiitake Pot Stickers

Prep time: 15 minutes | Cook time: 20 minutes | Makes 25 pot stickers

Dipping Sauce:	(optional)
¼ cup gluten-free tamari soy	1 medium shallot, fine diced
sauce	1 cup thinly sliced shiitake
2 tablespoons pure maple	mushrooms
syrup (optional)	2 cups sliced Brussels
½-inch piece of fresh ginger,	sprouts
peeled and finely grated	1 clove garlic, minced
1 green onion, finely sliced	1 piece of fresh ginger,
2 teaspoons sesame seeds	peeled and minced
Pot Stickers:	Salt and pepper, to taste
1 tablespoon virgin olive	(optional)
oil, plus extra for cooking	25 wonton wrappers

1. Make the Dipping Sauce: Whisk the tamari, maple syrup, ginger, green onion, and sesame seeds together in a small bowl. Set aside. 2. Make the Pot Stickers: Heat the olive oil in a large sauté pan over medium heat. Add the shallots. Stir and cook until fragrant and translucent, about 3 minutes. Add the shiitake mushrooms. Stir and sauté the mushrooms until they start to soften, about 2 minutes. Add the Brussels sprouts, garlic, and ginger, and stir. Season everything with salt and pepper, if using. Keep stirring the filling until the Brussels sprouts are bright green and slightly wilted, about 1 minute. Remove from the heat, and allow the filling to cool slightly. 3. Set out a small bowl of water. To assemble the pot stickers, divide the vegetable filling among the wonton wrappers, placing about 1 tablespoon of the filling in the center of each wonton wrapper. Take one filled wonton wrapper and dip your finger in the bowl of water. Moisten two sides of the wrapper, fold all sides together, and pinch along the edge to form a seal. Repeat with the remaining filled wrappers. 4. Wipe the sauté pan and heat a thin slick of olive oil over medium heat. Fry the pot stickers in batches until they're golden brown on all sides, about 1 full minute per side. Add more oil to the pan as needed to finish cooking all the pot stickers. 5. Serve the pot stickers hot with the dipping sauce on the side.

Per Serving:

calories: 42 | fat: 1g | protein: 1g | carbs: 8g | fiber: 1g

Baked Spaghetti Squash with Swiss Chard

Prep time: 15 minutes | Cook time: 55 minutes | Serves 4

2 small spaghetti squash	diced small
(about 1 pound / 454 g each),	4 cloves garlic, peeled and
halved	minced
Salt and freshly ground	2 teaspoons ground cumin
black pepper, to taste	2 teaspoons ground
1 large bunch red-ribbed	coriander
Swiss chard	½ teaspoon paprika
1 medium yellow onion,	½ teaspoon crushed red
peeled and diced small	pepper flakes
1 red bell pepper, seeded and	Zest and juice of 1 lemon

1. Preheat the oven to 350ºF (180ºC). 2. Season the cut sides of the squash with salt and pepper. Place the squash halves, cut side down, on a rimmed baking sheet. Add ½ cup of water to the pan and bake the squash for 45 to 55 minutes, or until very tender (the squash is done when it can be easily pierced with a knife). 3. While the squash is baking, remove the stems from the chard and chop them. Chop the leaves into bite-size pieces and set them aside. Place the onion, red pepper, and chard stems in a large saucepan and sauté over medium heat for 5 minutes. Add water 1 to 2 tablespoons at a time to keep the vegetables from sticking to the pan. Add the garlic, cumin, coriander, paprika, and crushed red pepper flakes and cook for 3 minutes. Add the chard leaves and lemon zest and juice. Season with salt and pepper and cook until the chard is wilted, about 5 minutes. Remove from the heat. 4. When the squash is finished baking, scoop out the flesh (it should come away looking like noodles) and stir it into the warm chard mixture.

Per Serving:

calories: 36 | fat: 0g | protein: 1g | carbs: 7g | fiber: 1g

Sweet and Savory Root Veggies and Butternut Squash

Prep time: 20 minutes | Cook time: 3½ to 5 hours | Serves 4 to 6

1 large sweet potato (about ½ pound / 227 g), peeled and cut into 1½-inch chunks

2 red or yellow potatoes (about ⅔ pound / 272 g), unpeeled and cut into 1½-inch chunks

1 medium yam (about ⅓ pound / 136 g), scrubbed, peeled, and cut into 1½-inch chunks

1 small butternut squash (about 1 pound / 454 g), peeled and cut into 1½-inch chunks

1 medium onion, diced

1 teaspoon ground ginger

4 carrots, cut into 1-inch rounds

2 apples, any variety, peeled and cut into 1-inch chunks

½ cup golden raisins

½ cup pitted dates, quartered

¼ cup maple syrup or date syrup (optional)

Juice from 2 oranges (about 1 cup)

Zest from 1 orange

1 cup store-bought low-sodium vegetable broth

2 teaspoons ground cinnamon

1. Place sweet potato, potatoes, yam, butternut squash, onion, carrots, apples, raisins, dates, maple syrup (if using), orange juice, orange zest, vegetable broth, cinnamon, and ginger in the slow cooker. 2. Cover and cook on High for 3½ to 5 hours or on Low for 8 to 10 hours, until the vegetables are tender and flavorful. Enjoy the delightful combination of sweet and savory flavors in this hearty dish!

Per Serving:

calories: 460 | fat: 1g | protein: 7g | carbs: 116g | fiber: 15g

Chapter 8 Desserts

Two-Ingredient Peanut Butter Fudge

Prep time: 5 minutes | Cook time: 5 minutes | Serves 8

1 cup chocolate chips	Sea salt (optional)
½ cup natural peanut butter	

1. In a small saucepan over medium-low heat, combine the chocolate chips and peanut butter. Stir often until the chocolate is melted and the mixture is well combined, approximately 5 minutes. Transfer the mixture into a pie plate or small glass container lined with parchment paper. If desired, sprinkle with sea salt for added flavor. 2. Refrigerate the mixture until it sets, for at least 1 hour or overnight. Once firm, slice the fudge into squares and serve. Store any leftovers in the refrigerator for up to 1 week. Enjoy the creamy and delicious peanut butter fudge!

Per Serving:

calories: 194 | fat: 12g | protein: 6g | carbs: 21g | fiber: 2g

Caramel-Coconut Frosted Brownies

Prep time: 10 minutes | Cook time: 25 minutes | Makes 12 brownies

Brownies:	Pinch ground cinnamon
1 (15-ounce / 425-g) can black beans, drained and rinsed	Frosting:
	1 cup pitted dates
½ cup rolled oats	6 tablespoons unsweetened plant-based milk
6 tablespoons pure maple syrup	2 tablespoons nutritional yeast
⅓ cup cocoa powder	¼ teaspoon vanilla extract
⅓ cup unsweetened applesauce	⅛ teaspoon red miso paste
2 tablespoons unsalted, unsweetened almond butter	¼ cup chopped pecans
	3 tablespoons unsweetened coconut flakes
1 teaspoon vanilla extract	

1. Preheat the oven to 350ºF (180ºC) and line a 12-cup cupcake tin with liners. 2. In a food processor, blend beans, oats, maple syrup, cocoa powder, applesauce, almond butter, vanilla, and cinnamon until smooth. 3. Transfer the mixture to the prepared cupcake tin, starting with about 2 tablespoons per cup and evenly dividing the remaining mixture. 4. Bake for 20 to 22 minutes until the tops are crispy and a toothpick inserted into the center comes out mostly clean. Remove from the oven, take the brownies out of the tin, and let them cool on a wire rack for about 5 minutes. 5. Meanwhile, in a food processor, blend dates, milk, nutritional yeast, vanilla, and miso until mostly smooth. 6. Pulse in pecans and coconut until well mixed but with some texture remaining. 7. Spread 1 heaping tablespoon of the frosting onto each brownie and serve.

Per Serving:

calories: 235 | fat: 11g | protein: 10g | carbs: 30g | fiber: 12g

Vanilla Corn Cake with Roasted Strawberries

Prep time: 20 minutes | Cook time: 50 minutes | Makes 1 cake

¾ cup full-fat coconut milk	½ teaspoon ground turmeric (optional)
1 teaspoon fresh lemon juice	
1 cup cornmeal	½ cup plus 2 tablespoons pure maple syrup (optional)
1 cup whole spelt flour	
1 teaspoon lemon zest	½ cup coconut oil, plus extra to grease pan
1 tablespoon aluminum-free baking powder	
	1 teaspoon vanilla bean paste or pure vanilla extract
¼ teaspoon baking soda	
1 teaspoon fine sea salt (optional)	4 cups whole strawberries

1. Preheat the oven to 350ºF (180ºC) and grease a 9-inch round cake pan with coconut oil. Line the bottom with parchment paper and grease it lightly. 2. Whisk together coconut milk and lemon juice in a medium bowl and let it sit for 5 minutes to curdle. 3. In a large bowl, whisk cornmeal, spelt flour, lemon zest, baking powder, baking soda, sea salt, and optional turmeric. 4. Make a well in the center of the dry mixture, add maple syrup, oil (if using), vanilla, and coconut milk mixture. Gently mix until smooth. 5. Pour the batter into the cake pan and bake for 25 to 28 minutes until golden and a toothpick comes out clean. Let it cool. 6. Raise the oven temperature to 400ºF (205ºC). Cut strawberries and roast them on a baking sheet lined with parchment until juicy and jammy, around 20 minutes. 7. Serve slices of the corn cake with roasted strawberries on top. Enjoy!

Per Serving: (⅛ cake)

calories: 394 | fat: 20g | protein: 6g | carbs: 52g | fiber: 5g

Tropical Colada Frozen Pops

Prep time: 5 minutes | Cook time: 0 minutes | Makes about 6 pops

¾ cup canned coconut milk	or frozen
2 cups chopped fresh pineapple	½ cup unsweetened shredded coconut
1 cup chopped mango, fresh	

1. Blend all the ingredients in a food processor or blender until mostly smooth, with a few small chunks remaining for texture. 2. Pour the mixture into ice pop molds, leaving some room at the top for expansion. Place the molds in the freezer and allow them to freeze until solid.

Per Serving: (1 ice pop)

calories: 137 | fat: 9g | protein: 1g | carbs: 14g | fiber: 2g

Peanut Butter Nice Cream

Prep time: 5 minutes | Cook time: 0 minutes | Serves 2

3 frozen ripe bananas, broken into thirds	2 tablespoons defatted peanut powder
3 tablespoons plant-based milk	1 teaspoon vanilla extract

1. In a food processor, combine bananas, milk, peanut powder, and vanilla. 2. Process on medium speed for 30 to 60 seconds until the mixture reaches a smooth soft-serve consistency. Serve immediately.

Per Serving:

calories: 237 | fat: 3g | protein: 10g | carbs: 45g | fiber: 7g

Gluten-Free Vegan Waffles

Prep time: 15 minutes | Cook time: 15 minutes | Makes 8 waffles

1¼ cups unsweetened almond milk	baking powder
2 tablespoons plus 2 teaspoons ground flaxseeds	½ cup mashed bananas or ½ cup mashed squash
½ cup almond flour	¼ cup melted extra-virgin coconut oil, plus more for the waffle iron (optional)
1 cup gluten-free oat flour	
½ cup millet flour	
¼ cup brown rice flour	1 tablespoon vanilla extract
1 tablespoon aluminum-free	1 teaspoon raw apple cider vinegar

1. In a medium bowl, whisk almond milk and ground flaxseeds together and let it thicken for at least 10 minutes. 2. Preheat the waffle iron. In another medium bowl, combine almond flour, oat flour, millet flour, brown rice flour, and baking powder. In the flax mixture, add mashed bananas or squash, oil, vanilla, and vinegar, and stir well. Add the flour mixture and stir until just combined. Lightly brush the waffle iron with oil and scoop about a scant ½ cup batter onto it. Cook until golden, slightly longer than regular waffles. Remove and serve immediately or cool on a rack if making ahead. Repeat with remaining batter. Store cooled waffles in airtight containers in the refrigerator for up to 3 days or freeze for up to 3 months.

Per Serving: (1 waffle)

calories: 193 | fat: 10g | protein: 4g | carbs: 23g | fiber: 2g

Cacao Pudding

Prep time: 10 minutes | Cook time: 0 minutes | Serves 2

1 ripe avocado, halved and pitted	1 teaspoon pure vanilla extract
2 tablespoons cacao powder	Pinch of sea salt (optional)
1 tablespoon pure maple syrup (optional)	2 tablespoons hazelnuts, chopped

1. In a blender or food processor, combine avocado, cacao powder, maple syrup (optional), vanilla, and salt (optional). Purée until smooth and thick, scraping down the sides as needed. 2. Transfer the mixture to 2 bowls, cover, and refrigerate until ready to serve. Sprinkle each bowl with 1 tablespoon of hazelnuts. Enjoy your creamy and indulgent cacao pudding!

Per Serving:

calories: 267 | fat: 19g | protein: 3g | carbs: 22g | fiber: 8g

Peanut Butter Cookies

Prep time: 10 minutes | Cook time: 15 minutes | Makes 10 cookies

2 tablespoons ground flaxseeds	1 tablespoon baking powder
6 tablespoons cold water	1 cup natural peanut butter
¼ cup maple syrup (optional)	½ cup whole-wheat flour

1. Preheat the oven to 350ºF (180ºC) and line a sheet pan with parchment paper. 2. In a large bowl, mix ground flaxseeds with water to make "flax eggs" and let it gel for about 10 minutes. 3. Add maple syrup (optional), baking powder, peanut butter, and flour to the bowl. Mix well with a fork. 4. Place rounded tablespoons of the batter onto the prepared sheet pan. Flatten each cookie and create a crisscross pattern using the back of a fork. Bake for 13 to 15 minutes until they are firm and slightly golden. Enjoy your peanut butter cookies!

Per Serving:

calories: 409 | fat: 28g | protein: 14g | carbs: 33g | fiber: 5g

Coconut Chia Pudding

Prep time: 5 minutes | Cook time: 0 minutes | Makes 3 cups

1 pound (454 g) raw young coconut meat, defrosted if frozen, any liquid reserved	coconut water
	1 tablespoon vanilla extract
1¼ cups unpasteurized	6 tablespoons chia seeds

1. In an upright blender, combine coconut meat (and any liquid if frozen), coconut water, and vanilla. Blend on high speed until smooth. Pour the mixture into a wide-mouthed quart jar or medium bowl. Add chia seeds and whisk thoroughly to ensure there are no clumps. Allow it to sit for a few minutes, then whisk again. Keep the whisk in place and refrigerate for at least 1 hour until completely chilled, whisking occasionally to distribute the chia seeds evenly. The pudding will thicken further overnight. If it becomes too thick, stir in a splash of water, coconut water, or nut milk. Store the pudding in an airtight glass jar or container in the fridge for up to 3 days.

Per Serving: (½ cup)

calories: 296 | fat: 26g | protein: 3g | carbs: 15g | fiber: 8g

Whole Wheat Berry Muffins

Prep time: 5 minutes | Cook time: 26 minutes | Makes 12 muffins

⅔ cup unsweetened plant-based milk	¼ teaspoon baking soda
1 tablespoon ground flaxseeds	¾ teaspoon salt (optional)
1 teaspoon apple cider vinegar	½ cup unsweetened applesauce
2 cups whole wheat pastry flour	½ cup 100% pure maple syrup (optional)
2 teaspoons baking powder	1½ teaspoons pure vanilla extract
	1 cup berries

1. Preheat the oven to 350ºF (180ºC) and prepare a 12-cup muffin pan with silicone liners or use a nonstick/silicone pan. 2. In a large measuring cup, vigorously mix plant-based milk, flaxseeds, and vinegar with a fork for about a minute until foamy. Set aside. 3. In a medium mixing bowl, sift together flour, baking powder, baking soda, and salt (if using). Create a well in the center and pour in the milk mixture. Add applesauce, maple syrup (if using), and vanilla, then stir together the wet ingredients in the well. Gently incorporate the dry ingredients into the wet ingredients until just moistened (avoid overmixing). Fold in the berries. 4. Fill each muffin cup three-quarters full and bake for 22 to 26 minutes, or until a knife inserted into the center of a muffin comes out clean. 5. Allow the muffins to cool completely for about 20 minutes, then carefully run a knife around the edges of each muffin to remove them from the pan.

Per Serving:

calories:124 | fat: 0g | protein: 3g | carbs: 23g | fiber: 2g

Almond-Date Energy Bites

Prep time: 5 minutes | Cook time: 0 minutes | Makes 24 bites

1 cup dates, pitted	¾ cup ground almonds
1 cup unsweetened shredded coconut	¼ cup cocoa nibs or nondairy chocolate chips
¼ cup chia seeds	

1. Blend all the ingredients in a food processor until crumbly and sticking together, scraping down the sides as needed. If you don't have a food processor, you can mash soft Medjool dates by hand. For harder baking dates, soak them first and then try blending in a blender. 2. Shape the mixture into 24 balls and place them on a baking sheet lined with parchment or waxed paper. Refrigerate for about 15 minutes to allow them to set.

Per Serving: (1 bite)

calories: 53 | fat: 3g | protein: 0g | carbs: 6g | fiber: 1g

Pumpkin Bread Pudding

Prep time: 10 minutes | Cook time: 25 minutes | Serves 8

1¼ cups pumpkin purée (a little over ½ of a 15-ounce / 425-g can)	½ teaspoon ground cinnamon
1 cup unsweetened plant-based milk	¾ teaspoon ground ginger
½ cup 100% maple syrup (optional)	¼ teaspoon ground nutmeg
2 teaspoons pure vanilla extract	¼ teaspoon ground allspice
2 tablespoons cornstarch	⅛ teaspoon ground cloves
½ teaspoon salt (optional)	8 slices stale whole wheat bread, cut into 1-inch cubes (about 6 cups)
	½ cup golden raisins

1. Preheat the oven to 350ºF (180ºC). Have ready an 8 × 8-inch nonstick or silicone baking pan. 2. In a large bowl, whisk together the pumpkin purée, plant-based milk, maple syrup (if using), and vanilla. Add the cornstarch, salt (if using), cinnamon, ginger, nutmeg, allspice, and cloves and whisk well. Stir in the bread cubes and raisins, and toss to coat completely. 3. Transfer the mixture to the prepared pan. Bake for 25 minutes, or until the top is golden brown and firm to the touch. Serve warm.

Per Serving:

calories: 192 | fat: 1g | protein: 4g | carbs: 31g | fiber: 2g

Nice Cream

Prep time: 10 minutes | Cook time: 0 minutes | Serves 2

2 cups frozen banana chunks	½ teaspoon vanilla extract
1 tablespoon soy milk	

1. Place bananas in a food processor and process until they become crumbly. 2. Add soy milk and vanilla to the processor. Process until the ingredients come together and form a texture similar to soft-serve ice cream. Serve immediately for a delicious and creamy treat!

Per Serving:

calories: 112 | fat: 1g | protein: 2g | carbs: 28g | fiber: 3g

Banana Bread Scones

Prep time: 15 minutes | Cook time: 20 minutes | Makes 10 scones

2 cups whole spelt flour	2 teaspoons pure vanilla extract
1 tablespoon aluminum-free baking powder	½ cup mashed ripe banana
1 teaspoon ground cinnamon	2 tablespoons hot water
½ teaspoon fine sea salt (optional)	⅓ cup chopped walnuts
⅓ cup pure maple syrup (optional)	⅓ cup Medjool dates, pitted and chopped
⅓ cup liquid refined coconut oil, plus extra for greasing the measuring cup (optional)	Serve: Coconut butter Jam

1. Preheat the oven to 350ºF (180ºC). Line a baking sheet with parchment paper, and set aside. 2. In a large bowl, whisk together the spelt flour, baking powder, cinnamon, and sea salt, if using. Make a small well in the center of the flour mixture and add the maple syrup, coconut oil, if using, vanilla, and mashed banana to the bowl. Gently stir the mixture with a spatula until the ingredients are slightly combined but there are still jags of flour throughout. 3. Add the hot water, chopped walnuts, and dates to the bowl and stir until everything is evenly combined. Avoid overmixing. 4. Lightly grease a ⅓ cup measuring cup with coconut oil. Scoop the scone batter up with the measuring cup and drop onto the prepared baking sheet with a little force. The portion of scone dough should come out in a nice puck shape. Repeat with remaining dough, spacing each scone 2 inches apart, and re-greasing the measuring cup if necessary. 5. Bake the scones for 20 minutes. Allow them to cool slightly on a wire rack before enjoying with coconut butter and jam.

Per Serving: (2 scones)

calories: 492 | fat: 21g | protein: 11g | carbs: 72g | fiber: 9g

Homemade Applesauce with Raisins and Nuts

Prep time: 10 minutes | Cook time: 25 minutes | Serves 6

6 medium apples, peeled, cored, and chopped	½ cup golden raisins
⅓ cup water	½ cup chopped pecans, toasted
¼ cup maple syrup (optional)	

1. Combine apples, water, and optional maple syrup in a large saucepan and bring to a boil. Reduce heat, cover, and simmer for 15 to 20 minutes until apples are tender. 2. Remove the lid, add raisins, and simmer for 5 more minutes to thicken. 3. Slightly mash the apples with a potato masher until chunky. 4. Top each portion with chopped pecans. Serve warm or chilled. Enjoy!

Per Serving:

calories: 233 | fat: 7g | protein: 2g | carbs: 46g | fiber: 6g

Nutty Raspberry Thumbprint Cookies

Prep time: 5 minutes | Cook time: 12 minutes | Makes 18 cookies

⅓ cup unsweetened applesauce	1¾ cups oat flour
¼ cup almond butter	½ teaspoon baking soda
½ cup date sugar (optional)	½ teaspoon salt (optional)
1 tablespoon ground flaxseeds	½ cup rolled oats
2 teaspoons pure vanilla extract	½ cup finely chopped walnuts
	⅓ cup raspberry jam, or to taste

1. Preheat the oven to 350ºF (180ºC) and line a large baking sheet with parchment paper or a Silpat baking mat. 2. In a large mixing bowl, beat together applesauce, almond butter, date sugar (if using), and flaxseeds until relatively smooth. Mix in the vanilla. 3. Add oat flour, baking soda, and salt (if using), and mix well. Fold in oats and walnuts. 4. Roll about 2 tablespoons of batter into a ball and place on the prepared baking sheet. Repeat with the remaining batter to make 18 balls. Moisten your thumb or index finger and create a deep indent in the center of each cookie. Fill each indentation with about ½ teaspoon of jam. 5. Bake for 10 to 12 minutes until the bottoms are golden brown. 6. Allow the cookies to cool on the baking sheet for 5 minutes, then transfer them to a cooling rack to cool completely.

Per Serving:

calories: 114 | fat: 5g | protein: 3g | carbs: 14g | fiber: 2g

Gluten-Free Vegan Muffins

Prep time: 10 minutes | Cook time: 35 minutes | Makes 10 muffins

¼ cup ground flaxseeds	coconut oil (optional)
1 cup unsweetened almond milk	¼ cup pure maple syrup (optional)
1 cup millet flour	¼ cup freshly squeezed orange juice
½ cup gluten-free oat flour	1 tablespoon vanilla extract
1 tablespoon aluminum-free baking powder	½ teaspoon fine sea salt (optional)
½ cup almond flour	Fruit, berries, or vegetables
⅓ cup melted extra-virgin	

1. Preheat the oven to 375°F (190°C) and line a standard muffin pan with 10 paper liners. 2. In a small bowl, combine ground flaxseeds and almond milk and let it thicken for 10 to 15 minutes. 3. In a medium bowl, sift millet flour, oat flour, and baking powder. Add almond flour and whisk to combine, breaking up any clumps. In another medium bowl, whisk together coconut oil, maple syrup, orange juice, vanilla, and salt (if using). Add the flax-almond milk mixture and whisk to combine. Stir in the flour mixture with a rubber spatula until just combined, adding any desired flavorings like fruit, berries, or vegetables. 4. Spoon the batter into the prepared muffin cups and bake for 35 minutes, or until a toothpick inserted in the center comes out clean. Allow the muffins to sit for 5 minutes before transferring them to a wire rack to cool completely. Store leftovers in an airtight container at room temperature for up to 2 days or in the fridge for up to 4 days. The muffins can also be frozen in an airtight container for up to 3 months. Thaw at room temperature in the container they were frozen in.

Per Serving:

calories: 212 | fat: 10g | protein: 4g | carbs: 27g | fiber: 3g

Almond Truffles with Toasted Coconut

Prep time: 10 minutes | Cook time: 0 minutes | Makes 8

¼ cup almond meal	2 tablespoons cacao powder
¼ cup toasted shredded coconut	2 tablespoons maple syrup (optional)

1. In a medium bowl, combine almond meal, coconut, cacao, and maple syrup (if using). Mix the ingredients with a fork or by hand until smooth. 2. Take about 1 tablespoon of the dough and roll it into a small ball. Repeat with the rest of the dough to make 8 truffles. 3. You can enjoy the truffles immediately or refrigerate them for 10 to 20 minutes before serving. These delicious treats are ready to delight your taste buds!

Per Serving:

calories: 42 | fat: 3g | protein: 1g | carbs: 5g | fiber: 1g

Gooey Bittersweet Chocolate Pudding Cake

Prep time: 15 minutes | Cook time: 3 to 4 hours | Serves 6 to 8

Cake:	2 tablespoons date syrup or maple syrup (optional)
1 cup whole-wheat flour	Nonstick cooking spray (optional)
¼ cup cocoa powder	Pudding:
2 teaspoons baking powder	¼ cup cocoa powder
½ teaspoon ground cinnamon	1 teaspoon instant coffee
¼ teaspoon salt (optional)	½ cup date syrup or maple syrup (optional)
⅓ cup unsweetened applesauce	1 teaspoon vanilla extract
2 teaspoons vanilla extract	1 cup hot water
⅔ cup unsweetened vanilla or plain plant-based milk	

1. Make the cake: In a medium bowl, whisk together the flour, cocoa powder, baking powder, cinnamon, and salt (if using). 2. In a separate medium bowl, whisk together the applesauce, vanilla, milk, and date syrup (if using). Pour the applesauce mixture into the flour mixture and stir until just fully combined. Do not overmix. 3. Coat the inside of the slow cooker with cooking spray (if using) or line it with a slow cooker liner. Add the cake batter and spread it over the bottom of the slow cooker. 4. Make the pudding: In a medium bowl, whisk together the cocoa powder, coffee, date syrup (if using), vanilla, and hot water. Pour over the cake ingredients in the slow cooker. The mixture will be watery. 5. Cover and cook on Low for 3 to 4 hours. When it is ready to serve, the cake will look dry on top and will have achieved a pudding-like texture below the surface. Enjoy it immediately for best results.

Per Serving:

calories: 195 | fat: 2g | protein: 4g | carbs: 44g | fiber: 4g

Zabaglione Cashew Cream

Prep time: 5 minutes | Cook time: 0 minutes | Serves 4

½ cup raw cashews	2 teaspoons lemon juice
½ cup apple juice	Fresh berries or other fruits, for serving
½ cup unsweetened raisins	

1. In a high-efficiency blender, combine the cashews, apple juice, raisins, and lemon juice. Blend until smooth. Transfer to an airtight container, and refrigerate until ready to serve. 2. To serve, put fruit in a bowl or dessert dish, and drizzle with the zabaglione.

Per Serving:

calories: 231 | fat: 8g | protein: 3g | carbs: 40g | fiber: 3g

Sweet Potato and Chocolate Pudding

Prep time: 10 minutes | Cook time: 0 minutes | Serves 4

2 cups cooked sweet potato, cooled	¾ cup unsweetened soy milk
1 cup pitted dates	6 tablespoons cocoa powder
	1½ teaspoons vanilla extract

1. In a high-efficiency blender, combine the sweet potato, dates, soy milk, cocoa powder, and vanilla. Blend until smooth, using a tamper accessory if necessary. Refrigerate in an airtight container until ready to serve.

Per Serving:

calories: 263 | fat: 2g | protein: 6g | carbs: 62g | fiber: 10g

Homemade Caramel with Dates and Peanut Butter

Prep time: 20 minutes | Cook time: 0 minutes | Serves 8

5 Medjool dates, pitted	2 teaspoons molasses
1 tablespoon peanut butter (no sugar or salt added)	8 small apples, cored and sliced into 8 wedges

1. Soak the dates in hot water for 10 minutes. 2. Drain the dates and place them in a food processor. Add the peanut butter and molasses and blend to a smooth consistency. 3. Refrigerate the caramel mixture for 20 to 30 minutes. 4. Serve 1 tablespoon of the caramel mixture with each sliced apple. Refrigerate the remaining caramel mixture for up to 5 days.

Per Serving:

calories: 145 | fat: 1g | protein: 1g | carbs: 36g | fiber: 6g

Poached Pears

Prep time: 10 minutes | Cook time: 20 minutes | Serves 2 to 4

2 cups apple juice	½ teaspoon vanilla extract
¼ cup unsweetened raisins	4 to 6 slightly ripe Bosc
½ teaspoon ground cinnamon	pears, peeled

1. In a large pan with a flat bottom, combine the apple juice, raisins, cinnamon, and vanilla. Place over high heat. 2. Quarter the pears. Using a melon baller, scoop out the seeds (or trim them out with a paring knife). 3. Add the pears to the liquid. Bring to a boil. Reduce the heat to medium. Partially cover, and simmer for 20 minutes, or until the pears are tender (a paring knife should easily slide into the pears). Remove from the heat. 4. Serve the poached pears with a drizzle of the cooking liquid.

Per Serving:

calories: 343 | fat: 2g | protein: 0g | carbs: 89g | fiber: 4g

Coconut and Tahini Bliss Balls

Prep time: 10 minutes | Cook time: 0 minutes | Makes 9 balls

½ cup cashews	(optional)
½ cups walnuts	3 tablespoons sesame tahini
½ cup rolled oats	½ cup unsweetened shredded
2 tablespoons maple syrup	coconut, divided

1. In a blender, pulse the cashews and walnuts until you have a combination of smaller pieces and nut dust. Transfer the mixture to a medium bowl and add the oats, maple syrup (if using), tahini, and ¼ cup of coconut and mix well. The mixture will be sticky. 2. Put the remaining coconut on a plate. Roll the mixture into 9 equal-size balls. Roll each ball in the coconut until evenly coated. Some will stick, some won't. It will only be a thin layer of coconut coating. 3. Set the finished balls on a sheet pan or plate and refrigerate for at least 30 minutes to set. Eat immediately or store in an airtight container and refrigerate for up to 7 days.

Per Serving:

calories: 419 | fat: 32g | protein: 10g | carbs: 29g | fiber: 6g

Quinoa Banana Muffins

Prep time: 10 minutes | Cook time: 24 minutes | Makes 12 muffins

2 cups spelt flour	peeled)
2 teaspoons baking powder	¼ cup plant-based milk
½ teaspoon baking soda	⅓ cup unsweetened
¾ teaspoon salt (optional)	applesauce
½ teaspoon ground cinnamon	2 teaspoons pure vanilla extract
½ cup date sugar (optional)	1 cup cooked quinoa,
1 cup mashed banana (from about 2 large bananas,	drained and rinsed until cool

1. Preheat the oven and line a muffin pan. 2. Sift dry ingredients, create a well, and mix in wet ingredients. Fold in quinoa. 3. Fill muffin cups and bake. 4. Allow muffins to cool and then remove from the pan. Enjoy these delicious and nutritious muffins!

Per Serving:

calories: 126 | fat: 0g | protein: 3g | carbs: 24g | fiber: 3g

Sweet Potato Spice Cake

Prep time: 5 minutes | Cook time: 45 minutes | Serves 6

1 sweet potato, cooked and peeled	1 teaspoon vanilla extract
½ cup unsweetened applesauce	2 cups whole-wheat flour
½ cup plant-based milk	½ teaspoon baking soda
¼ cup maple syrup (optional)	½ teaspoon ground cinnamon
	¼ teaspoon ground ginger

1. Preheat the oven to 350°F (180°C). 2. In a large mixing bowl, mash the sweet potato using a fork or potato masher. 3. Add the applesauce, milk, maple syrup (if desired), and vanilla, and mix well. 4. Stir in the flour, baking soda, cinnamon, and ginger until the dry ingredients are thoroughly combined with the wet ingredients. 5. Pour the batter into a nonstick baking dish or one lined with parchment paper. Bake for 45 minutes, or until a knife inserted into the middle of the cake comes out clean. 6. Allow the cake to cool, then slice and serve. Enjoy your delicious Sweet Potato Spice Cake!

Per Serving:

calories: 238 | fat: 1g | protein:5 g | carbs: 52g | fiber: 2g

Walnut Brownies

Prep time: 10 minutes | Cook time: 20 minutes | Makes 12 brownies

3 ounces (85 g) extra-firm silken tofu, drained	¾ cup water, heated until very hot but not boiling
⅓ cup pitted prunes, rough stems removed	2 teaspoons pure vanilla extract
½ cup unsweetened plant-based milk, heated until very hot but not boiling	1 cup whole wheat pastry flour
¾ cup 100% pure maple syrup (optional)	½ teaspoon baking soda
½ cup plus 2 tablespoons unsweetened cocoa powder	½ teaspoon salt (optional)
	½ cup walnuts, roughly chopped

1. Preheat the oven to 325°F (165°C). Line an 8 × 8-inch pan with a 10-inch square of parchment paper or have ready an 8 × 8-inch nonstick or silicone baking pan. 2. Crumble the tofu into a blender. Add the prunes. Pour in the hot plant-based milk and purée for about 30 seconds. Add the maple syrup (if using) and purée until relatively smooth. Some flecks of prune are okay, but there should be no chunks of tofu left. Scrape down the sides of the blender with a rubber spatula to make sure all the ingredients are incorporated. 3. Sift the cocoa powder into a mixing bowl. Add the hot water and mix with a fork until well combined. It should look like a thick chocolate sauce. 4. Add the prune mixture to the chocolate in the mixing bowl and stir to combine. Mix in the vanilla. 5. Sift in half of the flour and add the baking soda and salt (if using). Mix well.

Mix in the remaining flour and fold in the walnuts. 6. Spread the batter into the prepared baking pan. It will be rather thick, but you don't need to push it into the corners, as it will spread as it bakes. 7. Bake for 17 to 20 minutes. The top should be set and firm to the touch. 8. Remove the pan from the oven and let cool for at least 20 minutes. Slice the brownies into 12 squares and serve!

Per Serving:

calories: 148 | fat: 4g | protein: 3g | carbs: 26g | fiber: 2g

Salted Caramel Bites

Prep time: 5 minutes | Cook time: 0 minutes | Makes 18 bites

1 cup raw cashews	1 teaspoon pure vanilla extract
1 cup soft and sticky Medjool dates, pitted	¼ teaspoon sea salt (optional)
½ cup tahini	

1. In the bowl of a food processor fitted with the chopping blade, pulse the cashews until finely chopped. Add the dates and process until a thick, sticky paste forms. Stop to scrape down the sides of the bowl as needed. 2. Add the tahini, vanilla, and salt (if using) and process until the mixture forms a dough. If the mixture isn't sticking together well, add a tiny bit of water and process again. 3. Scoop out a heaping teaspoon of the mixture and roll into a ball about 1½ inches in diameter. Repeat to form approximately 18 balls. Freeze on a baking sheet until firm, then transfer to an airtight container and store at room temperature for up to 5 days.

Per Serving:

calories: 112 | fat: 6g | protein: 2g | carbs: 11g | fiber: 1g

Pistachio Protein Ice Cream

Prep time: 25 minutes | Cook time: 0 minutes | Serves 8

1 can low-fat coconut milk	Optional Toppings:
10 pitted Medjool dates	Pomegranate seeds
2 scoops organic pea protein	Fresh mint
1 tablespoon vanilla extract	Chopped dark chocolate
½ cup shelled pistachios	

1. Add all ingredients to a blender and blend into a smooth mixture. 2. Alternatively, add all ingredients to a medium bowl, cover it, and process using a handheld blender. 3. Freeze the mixture for 15 minutes, then stir it and freeze for another 10 minutes. 4. Add any desired toppings and freeze for at least 2 hours. 5. Store the ice cream in the freezer for a maximum of 90 days and thaw for 5 minutes at room temperature before serving.

Per Serving:

calories: 115 | fat: 4g | protein: 9g | carbs: 10g | fiber: 2g

Chocolate Chip Oat Cookies

Prep time: 10 minutes | Cook time: 15 minutes | Makes 20 cookies

¾ cup oat flour

¾ cup rolled oats

2 tablespoons hemp hearts or chia seeds

¼ cup pure maple syrup

3 tablespoons unsalted, unsweetened almond butter or other nut

butter

2 tablespoons tahini

1 tablespoon unsweetened soy milk

1 teaspoon vanilla extract

¼ cup vegan mini chocolate chips

1. Preheat the oven to 350°F (180°C) and line a baking sheet with parchment paper. 2. In a large bowl, combine flour, oats, and hemp hearts. 3. Add maple syrup, almond butter, tahini, soy milk, and vanilla, and mix thoroughly. 4. Stir in chocolate chips. 5. Drop 20 dough balls, about 1 tablespoon each, onto the prepared baking sheet, spacing them evenly. Gently press down to flatten the cookies. 6. Bake for 12 minutes or until the edges turn golden brown. Remove from the oven and let the cookies cool on the baking sheet for 10 minutes before transferring them to a wire rack to cool completely. Store in an airtight container.

Per Serving:

calories: 151 | fat: 8g | protein: 5g | carbs: 16g | fiber: 3g

Chapter 9 Stews and Soups

Spinach Vichyssoise

Prep time: 20 minutes | Cook time: 30 minutes | Serves 6 to 8

2 large leeks (white and light green parts), rinsed and diced

1 tablespoon chopped dill, or to taste

1 bay leaf

5 cups vegetable stock, or low-sodium vegetable broth

1½ pounds (680 g) russet potatoes (4 to 5 medium), peeled and diced

½ pound (227 g) spinach, chopped

Zest of 1 lemon

Salt and freshly ground black pepper, to taste

1 cup unsweetened plain almond milk

1. Place the leeks in a large pot and sauté over medium heat until tender, about 5 minutes. Add water 1 to 2 tablespoons at a time to keep the leeks from sticking to the pot. Add the dill and bay leaf and cook for another minute. Add the vegetable stock and potatoes and bring to a boil. Cook for 15 to 20 minutes, or until the potatoes are tender. 2. Add the spinach and lemon zest and season with salt and pepper. Cook for another 5 minutes, or until the spinach is wilted. Purée the soup using an immersion blender or in batches in a blender with a tight-fitting lid, covered with a towel. Return the soup to a pot and add the almond milk. Let cool completely, then chill until ready to serve.

Per Serving:
calories: 109 | fat: 0g | protein: 4g | carbs: 23g | fiber: 2g

Cauliflower, Chickpea, Quinoa, and Coconut Curry

Prep time: 15 minutes | Cook time: 3 to 4 hours | Serves 5 to 7

1 head cauliflower, cut into bite-size pieces (about 4 cups)

1 medium onion, diced

3 garlic cloves, minced

1 medium sweet potato (about ⅓ pound / 136 g), peeled and diced

1 (14½-ounce / 411-g) can chickpeas, drained and rinsed

1 (28-ounce / 794-g) can no-salt-added diced tomatoes

¼ cup store-bought low-sodium vegetable broth

¼ cup quinoa, rinsed

2 (15-ounce / 425-g) cans full-fat coconut milk

1 (1-inch) piece fresh ginger, peeled and minced

2 teaspoons ground turmeric

2 teaspoons garam masala

1 teaspoon ground cumin

1 teaspoon curry powder

Ground black pepper

Salt (optional)

½ bunch cilantro, coarsely chopped (optional)

1. In the slow cooker, combine cauliflower, onion, garlic, sweet potato, chickpeas, tomatoes, broth, quinoa, coconut milk, ginger, turmeric, garam masala, cumin, curry powder, pepper, and salt (if desired). 2. Cover and cook on High for 3 to 4 hours or on Low for 7 to 8 hours. When the cooking is complete, stir in the cilantro (reserving some for garnish) before serving each dish.

Per Serving:
calories: 503 | fat: 32g | protein: 11g | carbs: 48g | fiber: 12g

Deep Immune Cup of Soup

Prep time: 15 minutes | Cook time: 15 minutes | Serves 4

1 teaspoon virgin olive oil (optional)

1 small yellow onion, diced

1 medium carrot, diced

1 stalk celery, diced

3 cloves garlic, minced

1 (2-inch) piece of fresh ginger, peeled and minced

2 teaspoons turmeric powder

½ teaspoon dried chili flakes, to taste

⅔ cup whole-grain orzo

pasta or other small, shaped pasta

4 cups vegetable stock

2 teaspoons mellow or light miso

1 teaspoon apple cider vinegar

⅓ cup chopped fresh flat-leaf parsley

Salt and pepper, to taste (optional)

1. Heat the olive oil in a large pot over medium heat. Add the onions, carrots, and celery. Sauté and stir vegetables until the onions are very soft and translucent, about 5 minutes. 2. Add the garlic, ginger, turmeric, and chili flakes, and stir until the spices are fragrant, about 30 seconds. Add the orzo and vegetable stock. Bring to a boil. Lower the heat to a simmer, and cook until pasta is just tender, about 7 minutes. 3. In a small bowl, stir together the miso and apple cider vinegar. Ladle 2 to 3 tablespoons of the warm broth into the small bowl to fully dissolve the miso. Add this mixture to the soup along with the chopped parsley. Season the soup with salt and pepper at this point if you like. Serve immediately.

Per Serving:
calories: 83 | fat: 2g | protein: 2g | carbs: 16g | fiber: 3g

Split Pea and Sweet Potato Soup

Prep time: 5 minutes | Cook time: 40 minutes | Serves 4

2 cups dried split peas	2 large carrots, peeled and
1 tablespoon extra-virgin	cut into ¼-inch pieces
olive oil (optional)	1 teaspoon salt (optional)
2 garlic cloves, minced	2 sweet potatoes, peeled and
1 small yellow onion, diced	cut into 1-inch pieces
small	1 teaspoon ground turmeric
2 celery stalks, cut into	1 teaspoon smoked paprika
¼-inch pieces	

1. In a large pot, boil split peas with enough water to cover by 2 inches until they break down and form a thick gravy, about 30 minutes. 2. In a skillet, sauté garlic, onion, celery, carrots, and salt (if using) until fragrant and tender. 3. Add the sautéed vegetables, sweet potatoes, turmeric, and paprika to the pot. Cook, stirring often, until the sweet potatoes are fork-tender, approximately 10 minutes. Enjoy this comforting and nutritious soup!

Per Serving:

calories: 462 | fat: 5g | protein: 25g | carbs: 83g | fiber: 29g

Mushroom Barley Soup

Prep time: 10 minutes | Cook time: 40 minutes | Serves 4

1 cup pearled barley	diced small
4 cups water	1 celery stalk, minced
2 teaspoons extra-virgin	8 ounces (227 g) white
olive oil, divided (optional)	mushrooms, thinly sliced
1 small yellow onion, diced	1 teaspoon salt (optional)
small	¼ teaspoon dried thyme
3 garlic cloves, minced	½ teaspoon smoked paprika
2 large carrots, peeled and	

1. In a large pot, combine barley and water and bring to a boil over high heat. Reduce heat to medium-low and cook for about 40 minutes until tender. 2. While the barley is cooking, heat 1 teaspoon of olive oil in a large skillet over medium heat. Add onion, garlic, carrots, and celery and cook until vegetables are tender, stirring often for about 8 minutes. Add this mixture to the cooked barley. 3. Wipe the skillet clean with a paper towel and heat the remaining 1 teaspoon of oil over medium heat. Add mushrooms and cook, stirring occasionally, until browned, about 8 minutes. 4. Add mushrooms, salt (if desired), thyme, and paprika to the barley and vegetable mixture. Cook over medium heat, stirring often, until well combined and barley is soft, for about 20 more minutes. Spoon into bowls and serve hot.

Per Serving:

calories: 235 | fat: 3g | protein: 7g | carbs: 47g | fiber: 10g

Deconstructed Stuffed Pepper Stew

Prep time: 15 minutes | Cook time: 4 to 5 hours | Serves 6 to 8

1 medium onion, diced	1 (8-ounce / 227-g) can
1 medium red bell pepper,	tomato sauce
diced	4 cups store-bought low-
1 medium green bell pepper,	sodium vegetable broth
diced	1 tablespoon maple syrup or
2 celery stalks, diced	date syrup (optional)
1 cup brown rice	1 tablespoon Italian
1 cup dried green or brown	seasoning
lentils, rinsed and sorted	Ground black pepper
1 (14½-ounce / 411-g) can	Salt (optional)
no-salt-added diced tomatoes	

1. Combine onion, red bell pepper, green bell pepper, celery, rice, lentils, tomatoes, tomato sauce, broth, syrup (if using), Italian seasoning, black pepper, and salt (if using) in the slow cooker. Stir to mix, then cover and cook on Low for 4 to 5 hours. 2. After 2 hours, stir to prevent sticking. Continue to stir every 30 minutes until the rice and lentils are fully cooked. Enjoy your delicious Deconstructed Stuffed Pepper Stew!

Per Serving:

calories: 284 | fat: 2g | protein: 11g | carbs: 59g | fiber: 18g

Curried Acorn Squash Soup

Prep time: 20 minutes | Cook time: about 1 hour | Serves 6

1 acorn squash	broth
1 yellow onion, chopped	1 teaspoon curry powder,
2 garlic cloves, chopped	plus more for seasoning
2 celery stalks, coarsely	½ teaspoon dill
chopped	⅛ teaspoon cayenne pepper
1 tablespoon water, plus	1 (14-ounce / 397-g) can
more as needed	full-fat coconut milk
2 tablespoons whole wheat	Chopped scallions, green
flour	parts only, for serving
2 cups no-sodium vegetable	

1. Preheat the oven and bake halved acorn squash until tender. 2. Sauté onion, garlic, and celery in a pot. 3. Add flour, vegetable broth, roasted squash, curry powder, dill, and cayenne pepper. Simmer for 10 minutes. 4. Pour in coconut milk and blend until smooth. Serve topped with scallions and curry powder. Enjoy this flavorful soup!

Per Serving:

calories: 169 | fat: 13g | protein: 2g | carbs: 14g | fiber: 2g

Sweet Potato Bisque

Prep time: 20 minutes | Cook time: 40 minutes | Serves 6

1 large onion, peeled and diced
2 cloves garlic, peeled and minced
1 tablespoon grated ginger
1 tablespoon thyme
½ teaspoon ground nutmeg
1 teaspoon ground cinnamon
3 large sweet potatoes,
peeled and diced
6 cups vegetable stock, or low-sodium vegetable broth
Zest and juice of 1 orange
1½ cups unsweetened plain almond milk
Salt and freshly ground black pepper, to taste

1. Sauté onion in a large saucepan until softened. Add garlic, ginger, thyme, nutmeg, and cinnamon, and cook for another minute. Add sweet potatoes, vegetable stock, orange zest, and juice. Bring to a boil, then simmer covered for 25 minutes until sweet potatoes are tender. 2. Purée the soup with an immersion blender or in batches in a blender. Return to the pot, add almond milk, and cook for 5 minutes until heated through. Season with salt and pepper to taste. Enjoy this creamy and flavorful bisque!

Per Serving:

calories: 110 | fat: 0g | protein: 3g | carbs: 24g | fiber: 3g

Spinach, Barley and Carrot Soup

Prep time: 10 minutes | Cook time: 25 minutes | Serves 4

6 multicolored carrots, cut into 1-inch pieces
½ cup barley
1 (15-ounce /425-g) can diced tomatoes
2 garlic cloves, minced
4 cups no-sodium vegetable broth
2 cups water
4 cups fresh spinach
¼ cup chopped fresh basil
leaves, plus more for garnish
2 tablespoons chopped fresh chives, plus more for garnish
1 (15-ounce /425-g) can cannellini beans, rinsed and drained
1 tablespoon balsamic vinegar
Freshly ground black pepper, to taste

1. In a large pot, simmer carrots, barley, tomatoes with juices, garlic, vegetable broth, and water until barley is chewy. 2. Add spinach, basil, and chives on top, cover, and cook to soften leaves. 3. Stir in cannellini beans and vinegar, then let sit covered for 5 minutes. Garnish with chives, basil, and a pinch of pepper before serving. Enjoy this hearty and nutritious soup!

Per Serving:

calories: 261 | fat: 2g | protein: 12g | carbs: 50g | fiber: 14g

Tomato and Red Pepper Soup

Prep time: 20 minutes | Cook time: 30 minutes | Serves 4

2 medium yellow onions, peeled and coarsely chopped
2 large red bell peppers, seeded and coarsely chopped
3 large cloves garlic, peeled and minced
1 teaspoon thyme leaves
1 pound (454 g) fresh tomatoes (about 3 medium), coarsely chopped
Salt and freshly ground black pepper, to taste
¼ cup basil chiffonade

1. Sauté onions and red peppers in a saucepan. Add garlic and thyme and cook for another minute. 2. Add tomatoes and cook covered for 20 minutes. 3. Purée the soup until smooth using an immersion blender or blender. Season with salt and pepper. Serve garnished with fresh basil. Enjoy this delicious and comforting soup!

Per Serving:

calories: 55 | fat: 0g | protein: 2g | carbs: 12g | fiber: 2g

Minestrone

Prep time: 30 minutes | Cook time: 55 minutes | Serves 8 to 10

1 large onion, peeled and chopped
2 large carrots, peeled and chopped
2 celery stalks, chopped
4 cloves garlic, peeled and minced
8 cups vegetable stock, or low-sodium vegetable broth
2 tablespoons nutritional yeast (optional)
1 (28-ounce / 794-g) can diced tomatoes
2 teaspoons oregano
2 medium red-skin potatoes, scrubbed and cubed
4 cups packed chopped kale, ribs removed before chopping
½ cup uncooked brown basmati rice
6 cups cooked cannellini beans, or 3 (15-ounce / 425-g) cans, drained and rinsed
Salt and freshly ground black pepper, to taste
1 cup finely chopped basil

1. Sauté onions, carrots, and celery in a saucepan. Add garlic and cook for another minute. 2. Add vegetable stock, tomatoes, oregano, potatoes, kale, and rice. Simmer for 30 minutes. 3. Add beans and simmer for 15 minutes until rice is tender. Season with salt and pepper, and add basil for a delicious and hearty soup. Enjoy!

Per Serving:

calories: 118 | fat: 2g | protein: 5g | carbs: 24g | fiber: 7g

Vegetable Stock

Prep time: 10 minutes | Cook time: 1 hour | Makes 8 cups

1 tablespoon virgin olive oil (optional)	chopped
2 medium yellow onions, chopped and with papery skin left on	1 large leek
	4 cloves garlic, each cut in half
2 medium carrots, scrubbed and chopped	6 sprigs fresh thyme
	4 fresh parsley stems
1 parsnip, chopped	2 bay leaves
2 stalks celery, scrubbed and	7 whole black peppercorns
	8 cups filtered water

1. Heat olive oil in a large stock or soup pot and sauté onions, carrots, and parsnip until browned. Add celery, leek, and garlic, and continue sautéing until softened. 2. Add thyme, parsley stems, bay leaves, and black peppercorns to the pot, and deglaze with a splash of water. 3. Pour filtered water over the vegetables, bring to a boil, then simmer for 40 minutes. 4. Let the stock cool slightly, strain, and store in containers. Refrigerate for 5 to 6 days or freeze for up to 6 months. Enjoy the flavorful homemade stock in your favorite recipes!

Per Serving: (1 cup)

calories: 44 | fat: 2g | protein: 1g | carbs: 7g | fiber: 1g

Weeknight Chickpea Tomato Soup

Prep time: 10 minutes | Cook time: 25 minutes | Serves 2

1 to 2 teaspoons olive oil or vegetable broth	1 to 2 tablespoons balsamic vinegar or red wine
½ cup chopped onion	1 (19-ounce / 539-g) can diced tomatoes
3 garlic cloves, minced	
1 cup mushrooms, chopped	1 (14-ounce / 397-g) can chickpeas, drained and rinsed, or 1½ cups cooked
⅛ to ¼ teaspoon sea salt, divided (optional)	
1 tablespoon dried basil	2 cups water
½ tablespoon dried oregano	1 to 2 cups chopped kale

1. In a large pot, warm olive oil (if desired) and sauté onion, garlic, and mushrooms with a pinch of salt until softened, approximately 7 to 8 minutes. 2. Add basil and oregano, stirring to mix. Then, deglaze the pan by adding vinegar and using a wooden spoon to scrape up all the browned, savory bits from the bottom. 3. Add tomatoes and chickpeas, stirring to combine. Adjust the consistency by adding enough water. 4. Add kale and remaining salt. Cover and simmer for 5 to 15 minutes, or until the kale reaches your desired level of tenderness.

Per Serving:

calories: 272 | fat: 6g | protein: 13g | carbs: 45g | fiber: 14g

Miso, Lentil and Kale Soup

Prep time: 15 minutes | Cook time: 35 minutes | Serves 4

2 garlic cloves, minced	broth
2 small shallots, diced	1 tablespoon red miso paste
4 large carrots, thinly sliced	¼ teaspoon freshly ground black pepper
4 celery stalks, thinly sliced	
1 tablespoon water, plus more as needed	3 thyme sprigs
	1 cup dried brown lentils, rinsed
3 cups baby potatoes, halved and quartered	
	2 cups coarsely chopped kale
4 cups no-sodium vegetable	

1. In a large pot over medium-high heat, combine the garlic, shallots, carrots, and celery. Cook for 1 to 2 minutes, adding water, 1 tablespoon at a time, to prevent burning, until the shallots and celery start to become translucent. 2. Add the potatoes and cook for 3 to 4 minutes. 3. Carefully pour in the vegetable broth. Add the miso paste, pepper, thyme, and lentils. Bring the soup to a simmer, cover the pot, and cook for 15 to 20 minutes, or until the lentils and potatoes are tender. 4. Add the kale and cook for 3 to 4 minutes until wilted. 5. Refrigerate leftovers in an airtight container for up to 1 week or freeze for 4 to 6 months. The lentils will absorb some of the liquid; add more liquid or enjoy a thicker soup.

Per Serving:

calories: 292 | fat: 2g | protein: 15g | carbs: 58g | fiber: 12g

Lemony Herbed Lentil Soup

Prep time: 10 minutes | Cook time: 35 minutes | Serves 2

1 cup dried brown or green lentils, rinsed	1 potato, peeled and diced
	1 zucchini, diced
4 cups water	1 (15-ounce / 425-g) can crushed tomatoes
1 teaspoon extra-virgin olive oil (optional)	
	1 teaspoon Italian seasoning
½ small yellow onion, chopped	½ teaspoon smoked paprika
	2 cups baby spinach
2 garlic cloves, minced	Juice of 1 lemon
1 celery stalk, minced	1 teaspoon salt, plus more as needed (optional)
2 carrots, sliced	

1. Boil lentils in water until soft. 2. Sauté onion, garlic, celery, carrots, and potato in olive oil. 3. Combine with lentils, zucchini, tomatoes, Italian seasoning, and smoked paprika. Simmer to meld flavors. 4. Add spinach, lemon juice, and salt if desired. Stir until wilted and combined. Enjoy your flavorful Lentil Vegetable Stew!

Per Serving:

calories: 546 | fat: 5g | protein: 31g | carbs: 102g | fiber: 21g

Savory Squash Soup

Prep time: 20 minutes | Cook time: 27 minutes |
Serves 4

2½ cups butternut squash, peeled, halved, seeded, and diced (from about 1 medium)
1 large russet potato, diced (about 1 cup)
1 medium yellow onion, peeled and chopped (about ½ cup)
1 clove garlic, peeled and chopped

¼ teaspoon dried Italian herb mix, or a pinch each of oregano, basil, rosemary, and thyme
Pinch freshly ground black pepper, or to taste
¼ cup green peas
¼ teaspoon fresh lime juice
Finely chopped parsley

1. Bring 3 cups of water to a boil in a large pot over high heat. Add squash, potato, onion, garlic, herb mix, and pepper. Reduce heat to medium and cook covered for 20 minutes until vegetables are tender. 2. Use an immersion blender or regular blender (covered with a towel) to purée the soup. Return the soup to the pot and add green peas and lime juice. Cook for an additional 5 to 7 minutes until peas are tender. Serve hot, garnished with parsley.

Per Serving:

calories: 137 | fat: 0g | protein: 4g | carbs: 32g | fiber: 4g

Coconut Curry Soup

Prep time: 25 minutes | Cook time: 20 minutes |
Serves 6

3 tablespoons water
¾ cup diced red, white, or yellow onion
1½ teaspoons minced garlic
1 cup diced green or red bell pepper
1 (14½-ounce / 411-g) can diced tomatoes with their juices
1 (15-ounce / 425-g) can chickpeas, drained and rinsed

4 cups vegetable broth
1½ teaspoons ground cumin
2½ teaspoons curry powder
1 (13½-ounce / 383-g) can full-fat coconut milk
½ cup cooked brown rice
Salt and pepper, to taste (optional)
Optional Toppings:
Red chili flakes
Minced cilantro

1. Heat water in a large pot over medium heat. 2. Sauté onion, garlic, and bell pepper for 5 minutes until tender. 3. Add tomatoes, chickpeas, broth, cumin, and curry powder. Bring to a boil, then simmer for 10 minutes. 4. Stir in coconut milk and brown rice, cooking for an additional 5 minutes. 5. Season with salt and pepper to taste. Enjoy this flavorful and comforting soup!

Per Serving:

calories: 126 | fat: 2g | protein: 5g | carbs: 24g | fiber: 6g

Chickpea Noodle Soup

Prep time: 15 minutes | Cook time: 2 to 3 hours |
Serves 6 to 8

1 medium onion, diced
3 carrots, diced
3 celery stalks, diced
4 garlic cloves, minced
2 (14½-ounce / 411-g) cans chickpeas, drained and rinsed
8 cups store-bought low-sodium vegetable broth

1 teaspoon dried parsley
1 bay leaf
Ground black pepper
Salt (optional)
10 ounces (283 g) whole-wheat pasta spirals
Juice of ½ lemon
3 tablespoons chopped fresh parsley

1. Place onion, carrots, celery, garlic, chickpeas, broth, dried parsley, bay leaf, pepper, and salt if desired in the slow cooker. Cover and cook on High for 2 to 3 hours or on Low for 5 to 6 hours. 2. In the final 30 minutes of cooking, remove and discard the bay leaf. Add pasta and stir well. Check the pasta after 30 minutes for your preferred level of doneness. Stir in lemon juice and fresh parsley before serving.

Per Serving:

calories: 332 | fat: 4g | protein: 14g | carbs: 64g | fiber: 13g

Lentil Mushroom Soup

Prep time: 10 minutes | Cook time: 30 minutes |
Serves 4

⅔ cup dried green lentils
2 cups button mushrooms, sliced
1 red bell pepper
4 cups vegetable stock

¼ cup dried thyme
Optional Toppings:
Black pepper
Sun-dried tomatoes

1. Put a large pot over medium-high heat and add the vegetable stock along with the green lentils. 2. Bring the water to a boil and turn the heat down to medium. 3. Cook the lentils for about 15 minutes, without covering the pot, remove any foam produced by the lentils and stir occasionally. 4. Add the mushrooms and thyme to the pot, bring the heat down to a simmer, cover the pot with a lid and let it simmer for another 10 minutes. 5. Remove the stem, seeds and placenta of the bell pepper and dice the flesh. 6. Add the bell pepper to the pot, then make sure to stir well and let it simmer for another 5 minutes. 7. Turn the heat off and let the soup cool down for 5 minutes. 8. Divide between two bowls, serve with the optional toppings and enjoy! 1. Store the soup in an airtight container in the fridge, and consume within 2 days. Alternatively, store in the freezer for a maximum of 60 days and thaw at room temperature. The soup can be reheated in a pot or the microwave.

Per Serving:

calories: 146 | fat: 1g | protein: 10g | carbs: 24g | fiber: 12g

Tex-Mex Quinoa Vegetable Soup

Prep time: 20 minutes | Cook time: 3 to 8 hours | Serves 6

1 cup dried quinoa	1 (14-ounce / 397-g) can diced tomatoes
½ large yellow onion, diced	
2 garlic cloves, minced	1 (15-ounce /425-g) black beans, drained and rinsed
2 carrots, cut into coins	
2 celery stalks, cut into slices	1 (15-ounce /425-g) can red kidney beans, drained and rinsed
1 tablespoon water, plus more as needed	
¼ cup tomato paste	2 teaspoons chili powder
1 zucchini, cut into coins and quartered	1 teaspoon ground cumin
	6 cups no-sodium vegetable broth, plus more as needed
1 (14-ounce / 397-g) can whole-kernel corn, drained	

1. Place the quinoa in a fine-mesh sieve and rinse under cold water for 2 to 3 minutes, or until the cloudy water becomes clear. 2. On a 5-quart or larger slow cooker, set the temperature to High and let it heat for 5 to 10 minutes. 3. In the preheated slow cooker, combine the onion, garlic, carrots, celery, and 1 tablespoon of water. Cook for 2 to 3 minutes. Stir in the tomato paste to combine. 4. Add the zucchini, corn, tomatoes, black beans, kidney beans, chili powder, cumin, and vegetable broth. Stir well. The tomato paste will fully incorporate as the soup cooks. 5. Turn the heat to low. Cover the slow cooker and cook on Low for 6 to 8 hours or cook on High for 3 to 4 hours. If the soup seems too thick, add more broth or water, ½ cup at a time. 6. Refrigerate leftovers in an airtight container for up to 1 week or freeze for 4 to 6 months.

Per Serving:

calories: 334 | fat: 4g | protein: 16g | carbs: 62g | fiber: 14g

Caribbean Coconut Collards and Sweet Potatoes

Prep time: 20 minutes | Cook time: 35 minutes | Serves 4

1 tablespoon coconut oil (optional)	1 (15-ounce / 425-g) can red kidney beans or chickpeas, drained and rinsed
1 yellow onion, diced	
3 garlic cloves, chopped	1 (14½-ounce / 411-g) can diced tomatoes with juice
½ teaspoon crushed red pepper	
2 bunches collard greens, stemmed, leaves chopped into 1-inch squares	1½ cups water
	½ cup light or full-fat coconut milk
1 large sweet potato, peeled and diced	Salt and black pepper (optional)

1. Melt the oil (if desired) in a large, deep skillet over medium heat. Add the onion, garlic, and crushed red pepper and cook for 3 minutes. Stir in the collards and sweet potato, then add the beans, tomatoes with their juice, water, and coconut milk. 2. Bring the mixture to a boil, then lower the heat to medium-low. Cover the skillet and simmer for approximately 30 minutes until the collards and sweet potatoes are tender. 3. Season the dish with salt and pepper according to taste. 4. Serve the Caribbean Coconut Collards and Sweet Potatoes as desired.

Per Serving:

calories: 300 | fat: 12g | protein: 12g | carbs: 40g | fiber: 11g

Roasted Eggplant and Lentil Stew

Prep time: 20 minutes | Cook time: 1 hour 10 minutes | Serves 8

1 large eggplant	full-fat coconut milk
4 carrots, coarsely chopped	1 tablespoon red miso paste
4 cups no-sodium vegetable broth	1 tablespoon low-sodium soy sauce
1 cup dried brown or green lentils	1 (28-ounce / 794-g) can diced tomatoes
1 large yellow onion, diced	4 teaspoons ground cumin
1 bunch chopped scallions, white and green parts, divided	1 teaspoon adobo chili powder or smoked paprika
3 garlic cloves, diced	1 celery stalk, coarsely chopped
1 tablespoon water, plus more as needed	Fresh cilantro leaves, for serving
1 (14-ounce / 397-g) can	

1. Preheat the oven to 350°F (180°C). 2. Halve the eggplant lengthwise and place it on a baking sheet, flesh-side up. Spread the carrots around the eggplant on the same baking sheet. 3. Roast for 30 minutes, or until the eggplant and carrots are lightly browned or caramel colored and the carrots are fork-tender. 4. Set the carrots aside. Let the eggplant cool before handling it. Scoop out as much flesh as possible without scooping into the skin and set aside in a bowl. 5. In an 8-quart pot over high heat, bring the vegetable broth to a boil. Lower the heat to maintain a simmer and add the lentils. Cover the pot and cook for 20 to 30 minutes, or until the lentils are soft yet retain their shape. 6. While the lentils cook, in a small sauté pan or skillet over medium heat, cook the onion, white parts of the scallion, and garlic for 7 to 10 minutes, adding water, 1 tablespoon at a time, to prevent burning, until darkly browned. 7. In a blender, combine the roasted eggplant and onion mixture with the coconut milk, miso paste, and soy sauce. Purée for 2 to 3 minutes until smooth. 8. Once the lentils are finished cooking, add the tomatoes, cumin, chili powder, and celery. Bring the mixture to a simmer. Pour in the eggplant sauce and add the roasted carrots. Cook until warmed to your liking. 9. This stew is best served with a few fresh cilantro leaves and scallion greens on top.

Per Serving:

calories: 259 | fat: 10g | protein: 10g | carbs: 35g | fiber: 9g

Hot and Sour Soup

Prep time: 15 minutes | Cook time: 3 to 4 hours | Serves 6 to 8

6 ounces (170 g) shiitake mushrooms, sliced

1 (8-ounce / 227-g) can sliced bamboo shoots

4 garlic cloves, minced

1 (2-inch) piece fresh ginger, peeled and minced

1 (16-ounce / 454-g) package extra-firm tofu, drained and cut into bite-size cubes

8 cups store-bought low-sodium vegetable broth

¼ cup low-sodium soy sauce, tamari, or coconut aminos

¼ cup rice vinegar

½ teaspoon ground white pepper

½ teaspoon red pepper flakes

3 baby bok choy, chopped into bite-size pieces

2 tablespoons cornstarch

¼ cup water

4 scallions, green and white parts, chopped, for serving

½ bunch cilantro, chopped, for serving

1. Combine mushrooms, bamboo shoots, garlic, ginger, tofu, broth, soy sauce, vinegar, white pepper, and red pepper flakes in the slow cooker. Cook on High for 3-4 hours or on Low for 7-8 hours. 2. In the last 30 minutes, add bok choy. Mix cornstarch and water in a bowl and add the slurry to the slow cooker, stirring well. Serve the soup in bowls and top with scallions and cilantro. Enjoy the flavorful and comforting soup!

Per Serving:

calories: 138 | fat: 5g | protein: 11g | carbs: 14g | fiber: 4g

Roasted Red Pepper and Butternut Squash Soup

Prep time: 10 minutes | Cook time: 40 to 50 minutes | Makes 6 bowls

1 small butternut squash

1 tablespoon olive oil (optional)

1 teaspoon sea salt (optional)

2 red bell peppers

1 yellow onion

1 head garlic

2 cups water or vegetable broth

Zest and juice of 1 lime

1 to 2 tablespoons tahini

Pinch cayenne pepper

½ teaspoon ground coriander

½ teaspoon ground cumin

Toasted squash seeds (optional)

1. Preheat the oven to 350ºF (180ºC). 2. Prepare the squash for roasting by cutting it in half lengthwise, scooping out the seeds, and poking some holes in the flesh with a fork. Reserve the seeds if desired. Rub a small amount of oil over the flesh and skin, then rub with a bit of sea salt and put the halves skin-side down in a large baking dish. Put it in the oven while you prepare the rest of the vegetables. 3. Prepare the peppers the exact same way, except they do not need to be poked. Slice the onion in half and rub oil on the exposed faces. Slice the top off the head of garlic and rub oil on the exposed flesh. 4. After the squash has cooked for 20 minutes, add the peppers, onion, and garlic, and roast for another 20 minutes. Optionally, you can toast the squash seeds by putting them in the oven in a separate baking dish 10 to 15 minutes before the vegetables are finished. Keep a close eye on them. 5. When the vegetables are cooked, take them out and let them cool before handling them. The squash will be very soft when poked with a fork. 6. Scoop the flesh out of the squash skin into a large pot (if you have an immersion blender) or into a blender. Chop the pepper roughly, remove the onion skin and chop the onion roughly, and squeeze the garlic cloves out of the head, all into the pot or blender. Add the water, the lime zest and juice, and the tahini. Purée the soup, adding more water if you like, to your desired consistency. 7. Season with the salt (if using), cayenne, coriander, and cumin. Serve garnished with toasted squash seeds (if using).

Per Serving: (1 bowl)

calories: 58 | fat: 3g | protein: 1g | carbs: 5g | fiber: 0g

Lentil Chili

Prep time: 30 minutes | Cook time: 55 minutes | Serves 6 to 8

3 medium yellow onions, peeled and chopped (about 1½ cups)

1½ cups chopped celery

2 medium carrots, peeled and sliced (about 1 cup)

2 medium bell peppers, seeded and chopped (about 1 cup)

1 to 2 cloves garlic, peeled and minced

6 cups vegetable stock, or low-sodium vegetable broth

1½ tablespoons chili powder

1 teaspoon ground cumin

1 teaspoon paprika

½ teaspoon chipotle powder or smoked paprika

½ teaspoon cayenne pepper

2 cups red lentils, rinsed

1 (28-ounce / 794-g) can crushed tomatoes

1 (15-ounce / 425-g) can kidney beans, drained and rinsed

Zest and juice of 1 lime

Salt and freshly ground black pepper, to taste

1. In a large pot over medium-high heat, cook onion, celery, carrots, bell peppers, garlic, and 1 cup of vegetable stock until the vegetables soften, stirring occasionally for 5 to 7 minutes. Add chili powder, cumin, paprika, chipotle powder, and cayenne pepper. Cook for an additional minute, stirring well. 2. Add lentils, tomatoes, kidney beans, and remaining vegetable stock to the pot. Cover and bring to a boil over high heat. Reduce heat to medium-low and simmer, stirring occasionally, until lentils are soft, approximately 45 minutes. Stir in lime zest and juice, and season with salt and pepper.

Per Serving:

calories: 279 | fat: 1g | protein: 16g | carbs: 52g | fiber: 11g

Black Bean Soup

Prep time: 15 minutes | Cook time: 15 minutes | Serves 4

3 cups cooked or canned black beans	sweet corn
1 cup canned or fresh tomato cubes	4 carrots, sliced
	Optional Toppings:
4 cups vegetable stock	Jalapeño slices
1 cup cooked or canned	Fresh cilantro
	Lemon slices

1. If using dry beans, soak and cook 1 cup of black beans. 2. In a large pot over medium-high heat, add vegetable stock and black beans. 3. Bring to a boil, then simmer for about 10 minutes. 4. Add tomato cubes, corn, and carrot slices. Simmer for another 5 minutes, stirring well. 5. Turn off the heat and let the soup cool for 5 minutes. 6. Serve in bowls, optionally with toppings. Enjoy! 7. Store leftovers in an airtight container in the fridge for up to 2 days, or freeze for up to 60 days. Reheat in a pot or microwave before serving.

Per Serving:

calories: 233 | fat: 1g | protein: 14g | carbs: 41g | fiber: 14g

Lotsa Vegetable Chowder

Prep time: 30 minutes | Cook time: 30 minutes | Serves 4 to 6

8 small Yukon Gold, white, or russet potatoes (about 2 pounds / 907 g), cut into ½-inch chunks	1 cup chopped broccoli and cauliflower stalks, outer fibrous parts removed and discarded (about ½ pound / 227 g)
½ small onion, peeled and chopped	1 clove garlic, peeled and minced
3 ears fresh corn, kernels removed (about 1¾ cups), cobs reserved	2 tablespoons chopped thyme
2 medium carrots, peeled and diced	⅛ teaspoon white pepper
2 celery stalks, chopped	2 teaspoons ground cumin
¼ cup chopped red bell pepper	3 tablespoons chopped dill
	Salt, to taste (optional)

1. In a large pot, combine potatoes, onion, corn kernels and cobs, carrots, celery, red pepper, broccoli and cauliflower, garlic, thyme, white pepper, cumin, and 6 cups of water. Bring to a boil over high heat, then reduce to medium-low and simmer for 30 minutes until vegetables are tender. 2. Remove the corn cobs and let them cool. Take out 1 cup of the soup and blend it in a blender (cover with a towel) until smooth. If desired, blend 2 cups for a thicker soup. Return the puréed soup to the pot and add dill. Scrape the corn cobs with a knife to extract the creamy corn "milk" and add it to the pot. Stir well and season with salt if desired.

Per Serving:

calories: 262 | fat: 0g | protein: 8g | carbs: 60g | fiber: 6g

Zucchini Bisque

Prep time: 20 minutes | Cook time: 25 minutes | Serves 4

1 medium yellow onion, peeled and finely chopped	¼ teaspoon ground nutmeg
4 medium zucchini, finely chopped	½ teaspoon lemon zest
	½ to 1 cup unsweetened plain almond milk
2 cups vegetable stock, or low-sodium vegetable broth	Salt and freshly ground black pepper, to taste
½ teaspoon minced thyme	

1. Sauté onion in a large saucepan until tender. Add zucchini, vegetable stock, thyme, nutmeg, and lemon zest. Cook for 15 minutes until zucchini is tender. 2. Purée the soup with an immersion blender or in batches in a blender. Return to the pot, add almond milk, and season with salt and pepper. Heat until warmed through. Enjoy this creamy and delicious zucchini bisque!

Per Serving:

calories: 31 | fat: 0g | protein: 1g | carbs: 6g | fiber: 0g

Butternut Squash Soup

Prep time: 15 minutes | Cook time: 3 to 4 hours | Serves 5 to 7

1 medium onion, diced	diced
1 large carrot, diced	5 cups low-sodium vegetable broth or water, or enough to cover
1 celery stalk, diced	
1 Yukon Gold potato, unpeeled, diced	1 bay leaf
1 medium butternut squash (2 to 3 pounds / 907 g to 1.4 kg), peeled, seeded, and	1 teaspoon dried thyme
	Ground black pepper
	Salt (optional)

1. Place onion, carrot, celery, potato, and squash in a slow cooker. Add enough broth to just cover the vegetables (around 5 cups, depending on the size of the squash). Add bay leaf, thyme, pepper, and salt if desired. Cover and cook on High for 3 to 4 hours or on Low for 7 to 8 hours. 2. Remove and discard the bay leaf. Use an immersion blender or countertop blender to fully purée the soup before serving.

Per Serving:

calories: 101 | fat: 0g | protein: 3g | carbs: 25g | fiber: 6g

Chestnut Soup

**Prep time: 15 minutes | Cook time: 25 minutes |
Serves 4**

1 medium yellow onion, peeled and finely chopped	4 to 5 cups vegetable stock, or low-sodium vegetable broth
1 stalk celery, finely chopped	1 (15-ounce / 425-g) can chestnut purée
1 medium carrot, peeled and finely chopped	Salt and freshly ground black pepper, to taste
1½ tablespoons minced sage	
1 tablespoon minced thyme	2 tablespoons finely chopped parsley
1 bay leaf	
⅛ teaspoon ground cloves	

1. Place the onion, celery, and carrot in a large saucepan and sauté over medium heat for 15 minutes, or until the onion is tender and starting to brown. Add water 1 to 2 tablespoons at a time to keep the vegetables from sticking to the pan. 2. Add the sage, thyme, bay leaf, cloves, and vegetable stock. Bring the pot to a boil over high heat and whisk in the chestnut purée. Season with salt and pepper and cook for another 5 minutes. Serve garnished with the chopped parsley

Per Serving:

calories: 158 | fat: 1g | protein: 2g | carbs: 32g | fiber: 7g

Bean and Mushroom Chili

**Prep time: 20 minutes | Cook time: 38 minutes |
Serves 6**

1 large onion, peeled and chopped	½ teaspoon cayenne pepper, or to taste
1 pound (454 g) button mushrooms, chopped	1 tablespoon unsweetened cocoa powder
6 cloves garlic, peeled and minced	1 (28-ounce / 794-g) can diced tomatoes
1 tablespoon ground cumin	4 cups cooked pinto beans, or 2 (15-ounce / 425-g) cans, drained and rinsed
1 tablespoon ancho chile powder	
4 teaspoons ground fennel	Salt, to taste (optional)

1. Place the onion and mushrooms in a large saucepan and sauté over medium heat for 10 minutes. Add water 1 to 2 tablespoons at a time to keep the vegetables from sticking to the pan. 2. Add the garlic, cumin, chile powder, fennel, cayenne pepper, and cocoa powder and cook for 3 minutes. Add the tomatoes, beans, and 2 cups of water and simmer, covered, for 25 minutes. Season with salt, if using.

Per Serving:

calories: 229 | fat: 1g | protein: 14g | carbs: 42g | fiber: 15g

Hearty Chili

**Prep time: 10 minutes | Cook time: 10 to 20 minutes
| Makes 4 bowls**

1 onion, diced	1 (14-ounce / 397-g) can kidney beans, rinsed and drained, or 1½ cups cooked
2 to 3 garlic cloves, minced	
1 teaspoon olive oil, or 1 to 2 tablespoons water, vegetable broth, or red wine	2 to 3 teaspoons chili powder
	¼ teaspoon sea salt (optional)
1 (28-ounce / 794-g) can tomatoes	¼ cup fresh cilantro or parsley leaves
¼ cup tomato paste, or crushed tomatoes	

1. In a large pot, sauté onion and garlic in oil for about 5 minutes until soft. Add tomatoes, tomato paste, beans, and chili powder. Season with salt if desired. 2. Simmer the chili for at least 10 minutes or longer for better flavor development. Leftovers taste even better. 3. Garnish with cilantro and serve.

Per Serving: (1 bowl)

calories: 125 | fat: 5g | protein: 4g | carbs: 17g | fiber: 6g

Hearty Potato, Tomato, and Green Beans Stufato

**Prep time: 10 minutes | Cook time: 3 to 4 hours |
Serves 4 to 6**

1 large onion, chopped	salt-added crushed tomatoes
4 garlic cloves, minced	2 teaspoons dried oregano
3 red or yellow potatoes (about 1 pound / 454 g), unpeeled and cut into 1- to 2-inch chunks	2 teaspoons dried basil
	1 teaspoon dried rosemary
	½ teaspoon red pepper flakes (optional)
1 pound (454 g) fresh or frozen green beans, cut into bite-size pieces	Ground black pepper
	Salt (optional)
1 (28-ounce / 794-g) can no-	Chopped fresh parsley, for garnish (optional)

1. Place onion, garlic, potatoes, green beans, tomatoes, herbs, spices, and seasonings in the slow cooker. 2. Cover and cook on High for 3 to 4 hours or Low for 6 to 7 hours until potatoes are fork-tender. Garnish with parsley before serving. Enjoy this flavorful and comforting dish!

Per Serving:

calories: 197 | fat: 1g | protein: 8g | carbs: 40g | fiber: 9g

Chickpea Vegetable Soup

**Prep time: 15 minutes | Cook time: 30 minutes |
Serves 4**

1 yellow onion, coarsely chopped
2 carrots, coarsely chopped
2 celery stalks, coarsely chopped
1 red bell pepper, coarsely chopped
3 garlic cloves, minced
1 tablespoon water, plus more as needed
2 teaspoons grated peeled fresh ginger
1 small cauliflower head, cut into small florets
1 teaspoon ground turmeric
1 teaspoon Hungarian sweet paprika
6 cups no-sodium vegetable broth
2 cups chopped kale
1 (15-ounce /425-g) can chickpeas, rinsed and drained
Freshly ground black pepper, to taste
Chopped scallions, green parts only, for garnish

1. In a large pot over medium-high heat, cook onion, carrots, celery, bell pepper, and garlic for 5 minutes until the onion is translucent. Add water if needed to prevent burning. 2. Stir in ginger and cook for 30 seconds. 3. Coat cauliflower evenly with turmeric and paprika by stirring them into the pot. 4. Pour in vegetable broth and bring to a simmer. Reduce heat to medium-low, cover, and cook for 10 minutes. 5. Add kale and chickpeas, cooking for an additional 5 minutes to soften the kale. Season with pepper and garnish with scallions. 6. Store leftovers in an airtight container in the refrigerator for up to 1 week or freeze for up to 1 month.

Per Serving:
calories: 173 | fat: 3g | protein: 8g | carbs: 32g | fiber: 9g

Autumn Vegetable Stew with North African Spices

**Prep time: 35 minutes | Cook time: 50 minutes |
Serves 6 to 8**

1 large onion, peeled and chopped
2 large carrots, peeled and chopped
2 celery stalks, cut into ½-inch slices
3 cloves garlic, peeled and minced
1 tablespoon grated ginger
1½ tablespoons sweet paprika
2 teaspoons ground cumin
1 tablespoon ground coriander
2 (1-inch) pieces cinnamon stick
8 cups vegetable stock, or low-sodium vegetable broth
1 medium butternut squash (about 1 pound / 454 g), peeled, halved, seeded, and cut into ¾-inch pieces
1 turnip, peeled and cut into ½-inch pieces
1 russet potato, peeled and cut into ½-inch pieces
1 (15-ounce / 425-g) can crushed tomatoes
2 cups cooked chickpeas, or 1 (15-ounce / 425-g) can, drained and rinsed
2 large pinches saffron, soaked for 15 minutes in ¼ cup warm water
2 tablespoons finely chopped mint
Salt and freshly ground black pepper, to taste
½ cup finely chopped cilantro

1. Sauté onion, carrots, and celery in a large pot for 10 minutes. Add garlic, ginger, paprika, cumin, coriander, and cinnamon sticks and cook for 3 minutes. 2. Add vegetable stock, squash, turnip, potato, tomatoes, and chickpeas and bring to a boil. Reduce heat and cook for 25 minutes. Add mint and saffron, season with salt and pepper, and cook for 10 more minutes until vegetables are tender. 3. Serve the flavorful stew garnished with cilantro. Enjoy the warm and aromatic blend of North African spices in this hearty dish!

Per Serving:
calories: 156 | fat: 1g | protein: 6g | carbs: 31g | fiber: 6g

Indian Red Split Lentil Soup

**Prep time: 5 minutes | Cook time: 50 minutes |
Makes 4 bowls**

1 cup red split lentils
2 cups water
1 teaspoon curry powder plus 1 tablespoon, divided, or 5 coriander seeds (optional)
1 teaspoon coconut oil, or 1 tablespoon water or vegetable broth
1 red onion, diced
1 tablespoon minced fresh ginger
2 cups peeled and cubed sweet potato
1 cup sliced zucchini
Freshly ground black pepper, to taste
Sea salt, to taste (optional)
3 to 4 cups vegetable stock or water
1 to 2 teaspoons toasted sesame oil (optional)
1 bunch spinach, chopped
Toasted sesame seeds

1. In a large pot, boil the lentils with 2 cups of water and 1 teaspoon of curry powder. Simmer for about 10 minutes until lentils are soft. 2. In another pot, sauté onion and ginger in coconut oil (if using) until soft. Add sweet potato and cook for 10 minutes, then add zucchini and cook until shiny. Stir in 1 tablespoon of curry powder, pepper, and salt (if using). 3. Add vegetable stock, bring to a boil, then simmer and cover for 20 to 30 minutes until sweet potato is tender. 4. Add fully cooked lentils, pinch of salt, toasted sesame oil (if using), and spinach to the soup. Stir until spinach wilts, then remove from heat. 5. Serve with toasted sesame seeds as garnish. Enjoy!

Per Serving: (1 bowl)
calories: 238 | fat: 3g | protein: 15g | carbs: 38g | fiber: 9g

Quick and Easy Thai Vegetable Stew

Prep time: 20 minutes | Cook time: 20 minutes | Serves 4

1 medium yellow onion, peeled and diced small	1 (14-ounce / 397-g) can lite coconut milk
2 cloves garlic, peeled and minced	1 cup vegetable stock, or low-sodium vegetable broth
2 teaspoons grated ginger	3 cups mixed vegetables of your choice, such as edamame, water chestnuts, carrots, broccoli florets, or sugar snap peas
2 teaspoons Thai red chili paste, or to taste	
Zest and juice of 1 lime	
1 serrano chile, minced (for less heat, remove the seeds)	½ cup chopped cilantro
2 tablespoons low-sodium soy sauce, or to taste	2 tablespoons minced mint

1. Place the onion in a large saucepan and sauté over medium-high heat for 7 to 8 minutes, or until the onion is tender and starting to brown. Add water 1 to 2 tablespoons at a time to keep the onion from sticking to the pan. 2. Add the garlic, ginger, chili paste, lime zest and juice, and serrano chile and cook for 30 seconds. Add the soy sauce, coconut milk, vegetable stock, and mixed vegetables, reduce the heat to medium, and cook for 10 minutes, or until the vegetables are tender. Stir in the cilantro and mint and serve.

Per Serving:

calories: 336 | fat: 27g | protein: 5g | carbs: 21g | fiber: 7g

Moroccan Chickpea Soup

Prep time: 15 minutes | Cook time: 20 minutes | Serves 4

3 cups cooked or canned chickpeas	2 tablespoons Ras El Hanout
1 medium onion, minced	2 cups water
1 clove garlic, minced	Optional Toppings:
2 cups canned or fresh tomato cubes	Lemon slices
	Fresh cilantro
	Cranberries

1. When using dry chickpeas, soak and cook 1 cup of dry chickpeas. 2. Put a large pot over medium-high heat, and add the water, minced onions and garlic to the pot. 3. Bring the water to a boil then turn the heat down to medium. 4. Add the chickpeas and the Ras El Hanout spices and continue to cook for about 5 minutes, stirring occasionally. 5. After about 5 minutes bring the heat down to a simmer. 6. Add the tomato cubes, cover the pot with a lid and let it simmer for another 10 minutes. 7. Turn the heat off and let the stew cool down for 5 minutes. 8. Divide between two bowls, serve with the optional toppings and enjoy! 9. Store the soup in an airtight container in the fridge, and consume within 2 days. Alternatively, store in the freezer for a maximum of 60 days and thaw at room temperature. The stew can be reheated in a pot or the microwave.

Per Serving:

calories: 260 | fat: 2g | protein: 15g | carbs: 44g | fiber: 17g

Fiesta Soup

Prep time: 15 minutes | Cook time: 30 minutes | Serves 6

1 tablespoon avocado oil (optional)	1 (7-ounce / 198-g) can diced green chiles
1 yellow onion, diced	1 cup organic frozen corn
1 red bell pepper, diced	2 tablespoons fresh lime juice (from 1 lime)
1 zucchini, diced	
3 garlic cloves, minced	¼ cup fresh cilantro, chopped
2 tablespoons taco seasoning	
4 cups vegetable stock	Sea salt and ground black pepper, to taste
1 (15-ounce / 425-g) can black beans, drained and rinsed	For Serving:
	½ cup organic corn tortilla strips
1 (15-ounce / 425-g) can pinto beans, drained and rinsed	3 ripe avocados, diced
	½ cup fresh cilantro, roughly chopped
1 (15-ounce / 425-g) can organic diced tomatoes, undrained	1 lime, cut into wedges

1. Heat oil in a large pot over medium-high heat. Add onion and bell pepper, cook for 5 minutes until bell peppers start to brown and onions turn translucent. Add zucchini and garlic, cook for 1 more minute. Stir in taco seasoning and toast the spices for a bit longer. 2. Add stock, beans, tomatoes, and chiles. Bring to a boil, then simmer for 20 minutes until flavors blend and veggies become tender. Stir in corn, lime juice, and cilantro. Season with salt and black pepper. Remove from heat, ladle into bowls, top with tortilla strips, avocado, and cilantro. Serve with a lime wedge. Enjoy this flavorful and hearty Fiesta Soup!

Per Serving:

calories: 330 | fat: 18g | protein: 8g | carbs: 38g | fiber: 14g

Creamy Tomato Soup

2 carrots, coarsely chopped	1 tablespoon Hungarian paprika
½ cup water, plus 1 tablespoon and more as needed	1 (28-ounce / 794-g) can diced tomatoes
1 yellow onion, coarsely chopped	1 (14-ounce / 397-g) can full-fat coconut milk
2 to 4 garlic cloves, coarsely chopped	1 teaspoon dried thyme
1 (6-ounce / 170-g) can tomato paste	No-sodium vegetable broth or water, for thinning (optional)

1. In an 8-quart pot over medium-high heat, combine carrots and ½ cup of water. Cover and cook for 10 minutes until carrots are tender, adding more water if needed. Drain and set aside. 2. Place the same pot over medium-low heat and add onion and garlic. Sauté for 5 to 7 minutes, adding water 1 tablespoon at a time to prevent burning, until onion is browned. 3. Increase heat to medium-high and add tomato paste and paprika. Cook, stirring continuously, for 30 seconds to 1 minute. 4. Add diced tomatoes, coconut milk, thyme, and cooked carrots. Bring to a simmer, then cover and reduce heat to medium-low. Cook for 10 minutes, stirring occasionally. 5. Use an immersion blender to blend the soup until smooth. Alternatively, transfer the soup to a standard blender and blend in batches until smooth. 6. Thin the soup with vegetable broth or water as desired.

Per Serving:

calories: 292 | fat: 19g | protein: 6g | carbs: 28g | fiber: 7g

Chapter 10 Salads

Chickpea Apple Salad

Prep time: 15 minutes | Cook time: 15 minutes | Serves 2

1 cup cooked or canned chickpeas	1 large apple, peeled and cored
½ cup dry quinoa	Optional Toppings:
½ cup pomegranate seeds	Fresh mint
¼ cup tahini	Black pepper

1. If using dry chickpeas, soak and cook ⅓ cup of dry chickpeas as needed. Cook the quinoa for about 15 minutes. 2. Cut the peeled and cored apple into small pieces and set aside. 3. In a large bowl, mix the cooked chickpeas and quinoa. 4. Add the pomegranate seeds and apple pieces to the bowl and mix thoroughly using a spatula. Optionally, reserve some pomegranate seeds and apple pieces for garnishing. 5. Stir in the tahini until well combined with the chickpea and quinoa salad. 6. Divide the salad between two bowls and optionally garnish with the reserved pomegranate seeds, apple pieces, and a swirl of tahini. Add any optional toppings desired and enjoy! 7. Store the salad in an airtight container in the fridge and consume within 2 days. Alternatively, you can store it in the freezer for up to 30 days and thaw at room temperature. The salad can be served cold.

Per Serving:
calories: 234 | fat: 6g | protein: 11g | carbs: 32g | fiber: 6g

Greek Salad in a Jar

Prep time: 10 minutes | Cook time: 10 minutes | Serves 4

Salad:	too)
1 cup uncooked quinoa	Dressing:
1 cucumber, diced	¼ cup extra-virgin olive oil (optional)
2 cups cherry tomatoes, halved	½ cup fresh lemon juice
2 bell peppers, seeded and chopped	1 tablespoon Dijon mustard
½ cup walnuts, chopped	3 cloves garlic, minced, or 2 teaspoons garlic powder
¼ cup sun-dried black olives, sliced	¼ cup basil, finely chopped, or 1 tablespoon dried
4 cups chopped mixed greens (romaine is great,	1 tablespoon chopped fresh oregano, or 1 teaspoon dried

Himalayan pink salt and freshly ground black pepper	(about ¼ teaspoon each)

1. Cook quinoa according to package directions and let it cool. 2. Prepare the dressing in a small jar by combining all dressing ingredients, then shake to mix. 3. Assemble the salad in each jar by adding 1 to 4 tablespoons of dressing at the bottom. 4. Layer cucumber, cooked quinoa, tomatoes, bell peppers, walnuts, and olives. Finish with chopped mixed greens. 5. Seal the jar and store in the refrigerator for up to 4 days. 6. When ready to eat, pour the salad into a bowl, and the dressing will coat the ingredients. Toss gently if needed. Enjoy!

Per Serving:
calories: 399 | fat: 24g | protein: 10g | carbs: 39g | fiber: 6g

Pepperoncini Lentil Crunch Salad

Prep time: 15 minutes | Cook time: 25 minutes | Serves 8

Dressing:	Salt and pepper, to taste (optional)
4 pepperoncini peppers, stems removed	Salad:
2 tablespoons pepperoncini pickling liquid	2 cups French or black beluga lentils, rinsed
1 tablespoon white wine vinegar	1 red bell pepper, thinly sliced
1 clove garlic, chopped	1 small red onion, thinly sliced
½ teaspoon ground cumin	1 stalk celery, thinly sliced
½ teaspoon pure maple syrup (optional)	½ cup roughly chopped fresh flat-leaf parsley
¼ cup virgin olive oil (optional)	

1. Make the Dressing: In a blender, combine pepperoncini peppers, pepperoncini pickling liquid, white wine vinegar, garlic, ground cumin, maple syrup, olive oil, salt, and pepper (if using). Blend until creamy and smooth, then set aside. 2. Make the Salad: Boil lentils in a medium saucepan with water and a pinch of salt until tender, about 20 minutes. Rinse with cold water and transfer to a large bowl. 3. Add bell peppers, onions, celery, and parsley to the bowl. Season with salt and pepper (if using) and toss to combine. 4. Pour the dressing over the salad and toss once more. Serve immediately to preserve the crunch of the vegetables, and you can add extra pepperoncini peppers on the side. Enjoy!

Per Serving:
calories: 98 | fat: 7g | protein: 2g | carbs: 8g | fiber: 1g

Lentil Salad with Lemon and Fresh Herbs

Prep time: 10 minutes | Cook time: 45 minutes | Serves 4

1½ cups green lentils, rinsed	2 tablespoons finely chopped
3 cups vegetable stock, or	mint
low-sodium vegetable broth	4 green onions (white and
Zest of 1 lemon and juice of	green parts), finely chopped,
2 lemons	plus more for garnish
2 cloves garlic, peeled and	Salt and freshly ground
minced	black pepper, to taste
½ cup finely chopped	4 cups arugula
cilantro	

1. Place lentils in a medium saucepan with vegetable stock and bring to a boil over high heat. Reduce the heat to medium, cover, and cook for 35 to 45 minutes until lentils are tender. 2. Drain the lentils and transfer them to a large bowl. Add lemon zest and juice, garlic, cilantro, mint, green onions, salt, and pepper. Mix well. 3. To serve, divide arugula among 4 individual plates. Spoon the lentil salad on top of the greens and garnish with freshly chopped green onions. Enjoy!

Per Serving:

calories: 277 | fat: 0g | protein: 18g | carbs: 51g | fiber: 8g

Broccoli Caesar with Smoky Tempeh Bits

Prep time: 20 minutes | Cook time: 10 minutes | Serves 4

Creamy Cashew Caesar	1 bunch broccoli, cut into
Dressing:	florets
2 tablespoons raw cashew	1 teaspoon sweet paprika
butter	1 teaspoon smoked paprika
2 tablespoons filtered water	1 teaspoon pure maple syrup
1½ tablespoons fresh lemon	(optional)
juice	1 teaspoon apple cider
salt and pepper, to taste	vinegar
(optional)	½ teaspoon gluten-free
3 cloves garlic, grated	tamari soy sauce
1 teaspoon Dijon mustard	2 teaspoons virgin olive oil
1 teaspoon minced capers	(optional)
1 tablespoon nutritional	½ block (4 ounces / 113 g)
yeast	tempeh, crumbled
3 tablespoons virgin olive oil	Garnishes:
(optional)	2 teaspoons nutritional yeast
Salad:	Freshly ground black pepper
Pinch of salt (optional)	

1. Prepare the Creamy Cashew Caesar Dressing by combining the ingredients in a jar and shaking until smooth. Set aside. 2. Boil broccoli florets until tender and bright green, then drain and cool under cold water. 3. Mix paprika, smoked paprika, maple syrup, apple cider vinegar, and tamari in a small bowl. 4. Brown crumbled tempeh in a saucepan, then add the paprika mixture to coat the tempeh. 5. Arrange broccoli on a platter, drizzle with Caesar dressing, and top with smoky tempeh bits. Garnish with nutritional yeast and black pepper. Serve immediately.

Per Serving:

calories: 204 | fat: 19g | protein: 9g | carbs: 10g | fiber: 2g

Zingy Melon and Mango Salad

Prep time: 5 minutes | Cook time: 0 minutes | Serves 2

1 large mango, peeled,	into 1-inch pieces (about 2
pitted, and cut into 1-inch	cups)
pieces (about 1 cup)	Juice of 1 lime
½ small cantaloupe or	¼ cup chopped fresh cilantro
watermelon, peeled and cut	1 teaspoon chili powder

1. In a large bowl, combine the mango and cantaloupe. Add the lime juice and cilantro, and gently toss until well combined. 2. Spoon the salad into bowls and sprinkle with chili powder for an extra kick. Enjoy!

Per Serving:

calories: 171 | fat: 1g | protein: 3g | carbs: 42g | fiber: 5g

Pineapple Quinoa Salad

Prep time: 10 minutes | Cook time: 15 minutes | Serves 3

2 cups cooked or canned	1 red onion, minced
black beans	Optional Toppings:
½ cup dry quinoa	Chili flakes
1 cup fresh or frozen	Soy sauce
pineapple chunks	Shredded coconut
8 halved cherry tomatoes	

1. If using dry black beans, soak and cook ⅔ cup of beans as needed, and cook quinoa for about 15 minutes. 2. Combine all ingredients in a large bowl and mix thoroughly. 3. Divide the salad into 3 bowls, add optional toppings, and enjoy! 4. Store the salad in an airtight container in the fridge for up to 2 days or freeze for up to 30 days. Thaw at room temperature before serving. The salad can be served cold.

Per Serving:

calories: 310 | fat: 2g | protein: 16g | carbs: 56g | fiber: 14g

Tomato, Corn and Bean Salad

Prep time: 20 minutes | Cook time: 10 minutes | Serves 4

6 ears corn	and diced small
3 large tomatoes, diced	1 cup finely chopped basil
2 cups cooked navy beans,	2 tablespoons balsamic
or 1 (15-ounce / 425-g) can,	vinegar
drained and rinsed	Salt and freshly ground
1 medium red onion, peeled	black pepper, to taste

1. Bring a large pot of water to a boil. Add the corn and cook for 7 to 10 minutes. Drain and rinse the corn under cold water to cool. Cut the kernels from the cob. 2. In a large bowl, toss together the corn kernels, tomatoes, beans, onion, basil, balsamic vinegar, salt, and pepper. Chill the salad for 1 hour before serving.

Per Serving:
calories: 351 | fat: 2g | protein: 15g | carbs: 66g | fiber: 17g

Caramelized Onion Potato Salad

Prep time: 15 minutes | Cook time: 45 minutes | Serves 6

Dressing:	(optional)
3 tablespoons virgin olive oil	1 large onion, cut into ¼-inch
(optional)	slices
1 tablespoon grainy mustard	1½ pounds (680 g) mini new
1 teaspoon prepared	potatoes
horseradish	¼ cup chopped fresh dill
1 teaspoon raw agave	¼ cup lightly packed
nectar or pure maple syrup	chopped fresh flat-leaf
(optional)	parsley
1 tablespoon white wine	2 green onions, finely sliced
vinegar	⅓ cup chopped dill pickles
Salt and pepper, to taste	or bread-and-butter pickles
(optional)	Salt and pepper, to taste
Salad:	(optional)
2 teaspoons virgin olive oil	

1. Make the Dressing: In a jar with a tight-fitting lid, combine olive oil, grainy mustard, horseradish, agave nectar, white wine vinegar, salt, and pepper (if using). Shake the jar vigorously to combine and set aside. 2. Make the Salad: Heat olive oil in a large pot over medium-low heat. Add the onions and cook, stirring occasionally, for about 40 minutes until they are soft and deep golden brown. If the pan becomes dry, add a splash of water. Once caramelized, transfer the onions to a bowl and let them cool. 3. Meanwhile, boil the potatoes in a large saucepan with enough water to cover them by 1 inch. Simmer until just tender, about 15 minutes. Drain and cool the potatoes under cold water. Cut them into quarters,

wedges, or bite-sized pieces, and place them in a large bowl. 4. Add the cooled caramelized onions, chopped dill, parsley, green onions, and chopped pickles to the potatoes. Season with salt and pepper if desired. Pour the dressing over the potato salad and toss to combine. Serve the salad cold or at room temperature.

Per Serving:
calories: 180 | fat: 9g | protein: 3g | carbs: 24g | fiber: 3g

Refreshing Salad with Turnips, Apples, and Carrots

Prep time: 15 minutes | Cook time: 0 minutes | Serves 1

¼ cup raisins, no added	1 medium carrot
sugar	1 small turnip
1 medium apple	Pinch ground cinnamon
Splash freshly squeezed	(optional)
lemon juice	

1. Soak raisins in hot water for 5-10 minutes until softened. Let them cool. 2. Shred apple into a small mixing bowl using a box grater, including the juice. 3. Add a splash of lemon juice to prevent browning. 4. Shred carrot and turnip into the same bowl. 5. Add softened raisins and cinnamon (optional). 6. Mix well and enjoy.

Per Serving:
calories: 64 | fat: 0g | protein: 1g | carbs: 17g | fiber: 2g

Pinto Salsa Bowl

Prep time: 10 minutes | Cook time: 0 minutes | Serves 2

2 cups cooked or canned	¼ cup chopped fresh cilantro
pinto beans	Optional Toppings:
1 small Hass avocado,	Red onion
peeled, stoned, and cubed	Jalapeño slices
10 halved cherry tomatoes	Sweet corn
¼ cup lime juice	

1. If using dry pinto beans, soak and cook ⅔ cup of them. 2. In a large bowl, combine the cooked pinto beans with halved cherry tomatoes, avocado cubes, and chopped cilantro. 3. Add lime juice and stir thoroughly for even mixing. 4. Divide the pinto salsa between two bowls, garnish with optional toppings, and serve. Enjoy this delicious and nutritious bowl! 5. Store any leftovers in an airtight container in the fridge for up to 2 days or in the freezer for up to 30 days. Thaw at room temperature before serving.

Per Serving:
calories: 399 | fat: 10g | protein: 20g | carbs: 57g | fiber: 22g

Go-To Kale Salad with "Master Cleanse" Dressing

Prep time: 10 minutes | Cook time: 0 minutes | Serves 4

Dressing:	Salad:
2 tablespoons fresh lemon juice	5 cups packed chopped kale
1 tablespoon pure maple syrup (optional)	1 small fennel bulb, cored and shaved
3 tablespoons coconut oil (optional)	1 small sweet apple, cored and shaved
¼ teaspoon cayenne pepper	1 small shallot, peeled and shaved
Salt and pepper, to taste (optional)	¼ cup sunflower seeds, toasted, for garnish

1. Whisk together lemon juice, maple syrup, coconut oil, cayenne pepper, salt (if using), and pepper to make the dressing. 2. Place chopped kale in a large bowl and pour half of the dressing over it. Massage the dressing into the kale for about 3 minutes. 3. Add fennel, apple, and shallot to the bowl, and lightly toss with the kale. 4. Pour the remaining dressing over the salad, garnish with sunflower seeds, and serve immediately. Enjoy this refreshing and nutritious kale salad with its flavorful "Master Cleanse" dressing!

Per Serving:

calories: 229 | fat: 16g | protein: 5g | carbs: 22g | fiber: 5g

Creamy Potato Salad

Prep time: 10 minutes | Cook time: 20 minutes | Serves 4

5 large red or golden potatoes, cut into 1-inch cubes	½ tablespoon freshly squeezed lemon juice
1 cup silken tofu or 1 large avocado	½ teaspoon garlic powder
¼ cup chopped fresh chives	½ teaspoon onion powder
2 tablespoons Dijon mustard	½ teaspoon dried dill
	¼ teaspoon freshly ground black pepper

1. Bring a large pot of water to a boil over high heat. Immerse the potatoes in the hot water gently and carefully. Boil for 10 minutes or until the potatoes can be easily pierced with a fork. Drain the potatoes. 2. Transfer the drained potatoes to a large bowl and refrigerate for a minimum of 20 minutes. 3. In a separate large bowl, smash the tofu until creamy using a fork or mixing spoon. Whisk in the chives, mustard, lemon juice, garlic powder, onion powder, dill, and pepper until well combined. 4. Stir the cooled potatoes into the creamy dressing, ensuring they are well coated. Refrigerate the dish for at least 30 minutes or until ready to serve.

Per Serving:

calories: 341 | fat: 1g | protein: 10g | carbs: 74g | fiber: 12g

Slaw Salad and Avocado Dressing

Prep time: 15 minutes | Cook time: 0 minutes | Serves 6

Salad:	based milk
2 cups thinly sliced red cabbage	1 to 2 teaspoons minced garlic
1 cup grated carrots	1 to 2 tablespoons Dijon mustard
¼ cup packed chopped cilantro	½ tablespoon agave syrup (optional)
Dressing:	½ teaspoon salt (optional)
1 avocado, peeled and pitted	⅛ teaspoon freshly ground pepper
1 tablespoon lemon juice	
¼ cup unsweetened plant-	

1. In a large bowl, combine cabbage, carrots, and cilantro. 2. In a food processor or blender, blend avocado, lemon juice, milk, garlic, mustard, agave, salt (if using), and pepper until smooth. 3. Pour the avocado dressing over the salad and toss well to coat. Enjoy this creamy and nutritious slaw salad with a delightful avocado dressing!

Per Serving:

calories: 82 | fat: 5g | protein: 2g | carbs: 9g | fiber: 4g

Smoky Potato Salad over Greens

Prep time: 25 minutes | Cook time: 15 minutes | Serves 6

2 pounds (907 g) waxy potatoes	½ teaspoon salt (optional)
¼ cup apple cider vinegar	½ teaspoon smoked paprika
2 scallions, sliced	¼ teaspoon black pepper
1 teaspoon maple syrup (optional)	2 drops liquid smoke
1 teaspoon tomato paste	12 ounces (340 g) baby greens
½ teaspoon gluten-free Dijon mustard	¼ cup unsalted, roasted almonds, chopped

1. Steam or boil the potatoes in a large pot over medium-high heat until fork-tender, about 15 minutes. Drain and let cool in a single layer. 2. In a large bowl, whisk together the vinegar, scallions, maple syrup, tomato paste, mustard, salt (if desired), paprika, pepper, and liquid smoke. 3. Chop the cooled potatoes into bite-size pieces and add them to the bowl with the dressing. Gently toss to coat the potatoes. 4. Serve the potato salad over greens and top with almonds if serving immediately. If not serving immediately, refrigerate the salad for up to 5 days. Combine with the greens and almonds before eating.

Per Serving:

calories: 179 | fat: 3g | protein: 5g | carbs: 34g | fiber: 6g

Wedge Salad with Avocado Citrus Dressing

Prep time: 20 minutes | Cook time: 0 minutes | Serves 6

Dressing:
¼ cup filtered water
3 tablespoons fresh orange juice
3 tablespoons fresh lemon juice
2 tablespoons fresh lime juice
1 tablespoon apple cider vinegar
2 tablespoons raw agave nectar
3 tablespoons coconut oil (optional)
1 small jalapeño pepper, seeded and chopped
1 medium, ripe avocado, peeled and pitted

3 tablespoons chopped fresh dill
Salt and pepper, to taste (optional)
Salad:
3 romaine hearts, cut into wedges
1 head radicchio, cut into wedges
1 head Boston or Bibb lettuce, cut into wedges
Salt and pepper, to taste (optional)
2 cups cherry tomatoes, halved
Chopped fresh dill, for garnish

1. Blend water, orange juice, lemon juice, lime juice, apple cider vinegar, agave nectar, coconut oil, jalapeño, avocado, dill, salt, and pepper until smooth. Set aside. 2. Arrange romaine, radicchio, and Boston/Bibb lettuce wedges on a platter or plates. Season with salt and pepper. Pour the dressing over the wedges, and top with halved cherry tomatoes and chopped dill. Serve immediately. Enjoy this refreshing and flavorful salad!

Per Serving:

calories: 167 | fat: 12g | protein: 3g | carbs: 15g | fiber: 4g

Apple Broccoli Crunch Bowl

Prep time: 20 minutes | Cook time: 0 minutes | Serves 6

Bowl:
2 medium heads broccoli
3 diced apples
¼ cup diced red onion
½ cup raisins
½ cup sunflower seed kernels
¼ cup raw shelled hempseed
Dressing:

¼ cup cider vinegar
½ cup extra virgin olive oil (optional)
2 cloves garlic, minced
1 tablespoon maple syrup (optional)
½ teaspoon salt (optional)
¼ teaspoon ground black pepper

1. Cut the florets from the broccoli stalks and set aside the stalks. Cut the florets into very small pieces and place them in a large

bowl. 2. Remove the hard outer skin from the broccoli stalks to expose the tender inside. Discard the outer skin and cut the inside stems into matchsticks. Alternatively, use a mandolin or food processor with an appropriate attachment to cut the stems into long strips (not grated). The aim is to have small sticks of raw broccoli stems that will hold their shape. Add the matchstick-cut stems to the bowl along with the florets. Also, add the apples, onions, raisins, sunflower seeds, and hempseed. 3. In a separate medium bowl, whisk together all of the dressing ingredients until well combined. 4. Pour the dressing over the salad and toss everything together. Chill the bowl until ready to serve.

Per Serving:

calories: 296 | fat: 24g | protein: 9g | carbs: 18g | fiber: 4g

Chickpea Salad with Vegetables

Prep time: 5 minutes | Cook time: 0 minutes | Serves 1

1 cup canned chickpeas
1 small avocado, peeled, pitted, and sliced
1 medium tomato, diced
1 Persian cucumber, diced
¼ cup thinly sliced red onion
1 tablespoon freshly

squeezed lemon juice (optional)
1 tablespoon chopped cilantro
Pinch freshly ground black pepper
Pinch garlic powder

1. Drain the chickpeas. Place them in a medium mixing bowl. 2. Add the avocado, tomato, cucumber, and onion to the bowl. Drizzle with the lemon juice (if using). 3. Add the cilantro, pepper, and garlic powder. 4. Mix well and enjoy.

Per Serving:

calories: 636 | fat: 34g | protein: 20g | carbs: 72g | fiber: 28g

Creamy Fruit Salad

Prep time: 15 minutes | Cook time: 0 minutes | Serves 4

4 red apples, cored and diced
1 (15-ounce / 425-g) can pineapple chunks, drained, or 2 cups fresh pineapple chunks
¼ cup raisins

¼ cup chopped pecans or walnuts
1 cup plain plant-based yogurt
2 teaspoons maple syrup (optional)

1. In a large bowl, combine the apples and pineapples, ensuring the apples are covered in pineapple juice to prevent browning. Add raisins, nuts, yogurt, and maple syrup (if using), and mix well. Cover and refrigerate for at least 2 hours to develop flavors.

Per Serving:

calories: 267 | fat: 5g | protein: 6g | carbs: 54g | fiber: 6g

Quinoa Arugula Salad

Prep time: 10 minutes | Cook time: 20 minutes | Serves 4

1½ cups quinoa	1 red bell pepper, seeded and
Zest and juice of 2 oranges	cut into ½-inch cubes
Zest and juice of 1 lime	2 tablespoons pine nuts,
¼ cup brown rice vinegar	toasted
4 cups arugula	Salt and freshly ground
1 small red onion, peeled	black pepper, to taste
and thinly sliced	

1. Rinse the quinoa under cold water and drain. Bring 3 cups of water to a boil in a pot. Add the quinoa and bring the pot back to a boil over high heat. Reduce the heat to medium, cover, and cook for 15 to 20 minutes, or until the quinoa is tender. Drain any excess water, spread the quinoa on a baking sheet, and refrigerate until cool. 2. While the quinoa cools, combine the orange zest and juice, lime zest and juice, brown rice vinegar, arugula, onion, red pepper, pine nuts, and salt and pepper in a large bowl. Add the cooled quinoa and chill for 1 hour before serving.

Per Serving:

calories: 293 | fat: 6g | protein: 10g | carbs: 50g | fiber: 5g

Purple Potato and Kale Salad

Prep time: 10 minutes | Cook time: 15 minutes | Serves 4

5 to 6 small purple potatoes	1 clove garlic, peeled and
2 cups chopped kale	chopped
½ cup chopped tomatoes	¼ cup plus 2 tablespoons
1¾ teaspoons fresh lime	tahini
juice	½ teaspoon salt, or to taste
1 cup chopped cilantro, plus	(optional)
more for garnish	1 teaspoon cayenne pepper

1. Place the potatoes in a medium saucepan and add enough water to cover. Bring to a boil, reduce the heat to medium, and cook for 10 minutes, or until tender when pierced with a fork. Drain the potatoes and let them cool. Once cooled, peel if desired and cut into ½-inch cubes. 2. Place the kale and tomatoes in a skillet or saucepan and sauté for 2 to 3 minutes, or until the kale has softened slightly. Add water 1 to 2 tablespoons at a time to keep the vegetables from sticking to the pan. Add ¼ teaspoon of the lime juice and let cool. 3. In a blender, combine the cilantro, garlic, tahini, salt (if using), cayenne pepper, remaining 1½ teaspoons of lime juice, and 2 tablespoons of water. Blend until smooth. 4. To serve, prepare a bed of the cooked kale and tomatoes in a large salad bowl, top with the boiled potatoes, and spoon the dressing over the top. Garnish with chopped cilantro, if desired.

Per Serving:

calories: 261 | fat: 7g | protein: 7g | carbs: 43g | fiber: 7g

Curried Kale Slaw

Prep time: 20 minutes | Cook time: 0 minutes | Serves 4

Dressing:	to taste
⅔ cup water	Slaw:
2 tablespoons apple cider	1 apple, shredded
vinegar	1 tablespoon freshly
2 tablespoons pure maple	squeezed lemon juice
syrup (optional)	3 cups thinly sliced kale
1 garlic clove, minced	1 carrot, shredded
1 teaspoon grated peeled	1 cup shredded fennel
fresh ginger	¼ cup golden raisins
1 teaspoon Dijon mustard	¼ cup sliced almonds, plus
½ teaspoon curry powder	more for garnish
Freshly ground black pepper,	

Make the Dressing: 1. In a blender, combine the water, vinegar, maple syrup (if using), garlic, ginger, mustard, and curry powder. Season with pepper. Purée until smooth. Set aside. Make the Slaw: 2. In a large bowl, toss together the apple and lemon juice. 3. Add the kale, carrot, fennel, raisins, and almonds and toss to combine the slaw ingredients. 4. Add about three-quarters of the dressing and toss to coat. Taste and add more dressing as needed. Let sit for 10 minutes to allow the kale leaves to soften. Toss again and top with additional sliced almonds to serve.

Per Serving:

calories: 147 | fat: 4g | protein: 3g | carbs: 26g | fiber: 4g

Ancient Grains Salad

Prep time: 20 minutes | Cook time: 55 minutes | Serves 6

¼ cup farro	coarsely chopped
¼ cup raw rye berries	½ cup chopped fresh parsley
2 ripe pears, cored and	¼ cup golden raisins
coarsely chopped	3 tablespoons freshly
2 celery stalks, coarsely	squeezed lemon juice
chopped	¼ teaspoon ground cumin
1 green apple, cored and	Pinch cayenne pepper

1. Cook farro and rye berries in an 8-quart pot with enough water to cover by 3 inches. Boil, then simmer for 45 to 50 minutes until grains are firm but not hard. Drain and let cool. 2. In a large bowl, mix cooled grains with pears, celery, apple, parsley, raisins, lemon juice, cumin, and cayenne pepper. Serve immediately or store in the fridge for up to 1 week. Enjoy this wholesome and flavorful salad!

Per Serving:

calories: 127 | fat: 1g | protein: 3g | carbs: 31g | fiber: 5g

Blueprint: Classic Kale Salad

Prep time: 20 minutes | Cook time: 0 minutes | Serves 6

2 bunches kale, stemmed and chopped into bite-size pieces	spices(optional)
	2 cups shredded or chopped mixed crunchy vegetables
2 tablespoons gluten-free vinegar or citrus juice, plus more to taste	¼ cup finely chopped red onion, or 2 scallions, sliced
½ teaspoon salt, plus more to taste (optional)	Black pepper
	½ cup seeds or chopped nuts
¼ teaspoon dried herbs or	¼ cup dried fruit

1. Place the kale in a large bowl and drizzle with the vinegar, then add ½ teaspoon salt (if desired) and the herbs, if desired. Use your hands to massage the kale thoroughly, until it starts to darken in color and look slick. 2. Add the mixed vegetables and onion and toss to combine. Refrigerate for 8 hours or overnight, until ready to serve. 3. Just before serving, season with salt, pepper, and vinegar to taste and sprinkle with the nuts and dried fruit. Serve immediately or refrigerate for up to 3 days.

Per Serving:

calories: 125 | fat: 5g | protein: 6g | carbs: 17g | fiber: 5g

Taco Tempeh Salad

Prep time: 25 minutes | Cook time: 15 minutes | Serves 3

1 cup cooked black beans	¼ teaspoon cumin
1 (8-ounce / 227-g) package tempeh	¼ teaspoon paprika
	1 large bunch of fresh or frozen kale, chopped
1 tablespoon lime or lemon juice	1 large avocado, peeled, pitted, and diced
2 tablespoons extra virgin olive oil (optional)	½ cup salsa
1 teaspoon maple syrup (optional)	Salt and pepper to taste (optional)
½ teaspoon chili powder	

1. Cut the tempeh into ¼-inch cubes; then add the cut tempeh, lime or lemon juice, 1 tablespoon of olive oil, maple syrup, chili powder, cumin, and paprika to a bowl. Stir well and let the tempeh marinate in the fridge for at least 1 hour, up to 12 hours. 2. Heat the remaining 1 tablespoon of olive oil in a frying pan over medium heat. Add the marinated tempeh mixture and cook until brown and crispy on both sides, around 10 minutes. Put the chopped kale in a bowl with the cooked beans and prepared tempeh. 3. Store, or serve the salad immediately, topped with salsa, avocado, and salt and pepper to taste, if desired.

Per Serving:

calories: 441 | fat: 23g | protein: 22g | carbs: 36g | fiber: 18g

Spinach Salad with Sweet Smoky Dressing

Prep time: 15 minutes | Cook time: 0 minutes | Serves 4 to 6

Dressing:	½ teaspoon smoked paprika
¼ cup balsamic vinegar	Salad:
2 tablespoons soy sauce	4 to 6 cups spinach
3 tablespoons pure maple syrup	2 cups sliced strawberries
1½ tablespoons Dijon mustard	¼ red or white onion, thinly sliced and rinsed

Make the Dressing: 1. In a small bowl or container with a lid, combine the vinegar, soy sauce, maple syrup, mustard, and paprika. Whisk vigorously or shake. Make the Salad: 2. In a large bowl, combine the spinach, strawberries, and onion. 3. Add the dressing, and toss to coat. Serve immediately.

Per Serving:

calories: 84 | fat: 1g | protein: 2g | carbs: 18g | fiber: 3g

Crunchy Curry Salad

Prep time: 20 minutes | Cook time: 0 minutes | Serves 4

1 head napa cabbage	coconut milk
1 cup shredded carrots	¼ cup rice vinegar
1 red bell pepper, julienned	¼ cup diced yellow onion
½ cup thinly sliced scallions	2 tablespoons white miso paste
½ cup fresh cilantro, roughly chopped	2 tablespoons pure maple syrup (optional)
½ cup sunflower seeds	1 tablespoon red curry paste
1 jalapeño chile pepper, thickly sliced	1 garlic clove, minced
½ cup creamy almond butter	½-inch piece fresh ginger, peeled
¼ cup canned full-fat	

1. Trim the end of the cabbage, halve and core it, and cut into very thin ribbons, or shred. Place in a bowl with the carrots, bell pepper, scallions, cilantro, sunflower seeds, and chile pepper. Set aside. 2. In a blender, make a curry sauce by combining the almond butter, coconut milk, vinegar, onion, miso, maple syrup (if using), curry paste, garlic, and ginger and purée until smooth. Stop to scrape down the sides as needed. If the mixture is too thick, add a little more coconut milk and blend again. 3. Pour the sauce over the cabbage mixture. Toss well to combine. Serve immediately or store in an airtight container for up to 5 days.

Per Serving:

calories: 478 | fat: 31g | protein: 16g | carbs: 42g | fiber: 15g

Vegan "Toona" Salad

3 cups cooked chickpeas	1½ tablespoons freshly
1 avocado, peeled and pitted	squeezed lemon juice
½ cup chopped red onion	½ tablespoon maple syrup
¼ cup chopped celery	(optional)
2 tablespoons Dijon mustard	1 teaspoon garlic powder

1. In a large bowl, combine the chickpeas and the avocado. Using a fork or a potato masher, smash them down until the majority of the chickpeas have been broken apart. 2. Stir in the onion, celery, mustard, lemon juice, maple syrup (if desired), and garlic powder, making sure everything is thoroughly combined, and serve.

Per Serving:

calories: 298 | fat: 10g | protein: 13g | carbs: 42g | fiber: 13g

Mango Black Bean Salad

4 cups cooked black beans, or 2 (15-ounce / 425-g) cans, drained and rinsed	sliced
	½ cup finely chopped cilantro
2 mangoes, peeled, halved, pitted, and diced	1 jalapeño pepper, minced (for less heat, remove the seeds)
1 medium red bell pepper, seeded and diced small	½ cup red wine vinegar
1 bunch green onions (green and white parts), thinly	Zest and juice of 1 orange
	Zest and juice of 1 lime

1. Combine all ingredients in a large bowl and mix well. Chill for 1 hour before serving.

Per Serving:

calories: 299 | fat: 1g | protein: 16g | carbs: 56g | fiber: 17g

Roasted Root Vegetable Salad Bowl

Roasted Vegetables:	1 tablespoon lemon juice
1 sweet potato, peeled and chopped into bite-size pieces	1 clove garlic
1 parsnip, peeled and sliced into ¼-inch rounds	¼ teaspoon salt (optional)
	Pinch of ground black pepper
2 carrots, peeled and sliced into ½-inch rounds	3 tablespoons water
2 tablespoons extra virgin olive oil (optional)	Assemble:
	¼ cup diced red onion
½ teaspoon salt (optional)	½ cup chopped red cabbage
Tahini Dressing:	9 ounces (255 g) baby spinach
¼ cup tahini	¼ cup raw shelled hempseed
1 tablespoon maple syrup (optional)	1 tablespoon black or white chia seeds

Make Roasted Vegetables: 1. Preheat the oven to 375ºF (190ºC). 2. Place the sweet potatoes, parsnips, and carrots on a baking sheet, keeping them separated. Drizzle the oil (if desired) over the top and lightly toss, still keeping the vegetables separated. Sprinkle with salt, if desired. Bake for 30 to 35 minutes or until they can be pierced with a fork. Set aside. Make Tahini Dressing: 3. Add all the dressing ingredients to a blender and blend until smooth. Assemble: 4. Prepare the salad bowls by placing half the spinach in the bottom of each bowl. Arrange all the remaining vegetables and hempseed in a circle around the edge of the bowl. Pour half of the dressing in the center of the vegetable round. Sprinkle with the chia seeds.

Per Serving:

calories: 395 | fat: 22g | protein: 24g | carbs: 26g | fiber: 8g

Chapter 11 Staples, Sauces, Dips, and Dressings

Tahini-Maple Granola

Prep time: 10 minutes | Cook time: 40 minutes | Makes 2½ cups

1 cup rolled oats
¼ cup unsweetened raisins
¼ cup pecan pieces
¼ cup walnut pieces
¼ cup sliced almonds

¼ cup vegan chocolate chips
3 tablespoons tahini
3 tablespoons pure maple syrup

1. Preheat the oven to 350ºF (180ºC) and line a baking sheet with parchment paper. 2. In a large bowl, combine oats, raisins, pecans, walnuts, almonds, and chocolate chips. 3. Add tahini and maple syrup, mixing thoroughly. 4. Spread the mixture in a thin layer on the prepared baking sheet (for chunkier granola, leave some small chunks together). 5. Bake for 35 to 40 minutes at the preheated oven, stirring halfway through, until the granola turns crispy and golden brown. 6. Once done, remove from the oven and store in an airtight container for up to 1 week. Enjoy this delightful and nutritious Tahini-Maple Granola!

Per Serving:
calories: 145 | fat: 8g | protein: 4g | carbs: 3g | fiber: 2g

Coconut Butter

Prep time: 5 minutes | Cook time: 0 minutes | Makes 1 cup

4 cups unsweetened shredded dried coconut or 7 cups unsweetened flaked dried coconut

1. Place the coconut in a food processor and process for 10 to 15 minutes, making sure to scrape down the sides every few minutes. Continue until the butter becomes smooth and reaches a liquid consistency. 2. Transfer the coconut butter into a tightly sealed glass jar. Store it at room temperature, and it should remain good for up to 1 month. Enjoy the creamy and versatile coconut butter in your favorite recipes!

Per Serving: (½ cup)
calories: 280 | fat: 28g | protein: 3g | carbs: 10g | fiber: 7g

Cashew Cheese Spread

Prep time: 5 minutes | Cook time: 0 minutes | Serves 5

1 cup water
1 cup raw cashews
1 teaspoon nutritional yeast

½ teaspoon salt (optional)
1 teaspoon garlic powder (optional)

1. Soak the cashews in water for 6 hours in a medium-sized bowl. Drain the soaked cashews and transfer them to a food processor. Add 1 cup of water and all the other ingredients. Blend the mixture until smooth and creamy. 2. Enjoy the Cashew Cheese Spread immediately or store it for later use. For the best flavor, refrigerate the spread and serve it chilled. This delicious and versatile cheese alternative can be used as a spread, dip, or topping for various dishes!

Per Serving:
calories: 151 | fat: 11g | protein: 5g | carbs: 9g | fiber: 1g

Strawberry Chia Jam

Prep time: 2 minutes | Cook time: 10 minutes | Makes 1½ cups

3 cups frozen strawberries
4 dates, pitted and chopped small

¼ cup water
3 tablespoons chia seeds

1. In a medium saucepan over medium-high heat, combine strawberries, dates, and water. Bring the mixture to a boil, then lower the heat to medium-low and let it simmer for 10 minutes, stirring occasionally. Remove from the heat. 2. Use a potato masher to mash the mixture until the jam becomes smooth, while still leaving some chunks. Add chia seeds and stir well. Transfer the jam into a small jar, cover it, and let it cool. As it cools, the jam will thicken. Store the jam in the refrigerator for up to 5 days. Enjoy the delightful and nutritious Strawberry Chia Jam!

Per Serving:
calories: 43 | fat: 1g | protein: 1g | carbs: 8g | fiber: 3g

Jackfruit Carnitas Tacos

Prep time: 10 minutes | Cook time: 20 minutes | Serves 4

1 (20-ounce / 567-g) can young green jackfruit, drained	cinnamon
	1 teaspoon liquid smoke
½ cup diced red, white, or yellow onion	½ cup vegetable broth
	8 corn tortillas
1 teaspoon minced garlic	Optional Toppings:
3 tablespoons water	1 sliced avocado
1 tablespoon ground cumin	1 handful chopped cilantro
½ tablespoon ground coriander	Squeeze of lime juice
	Hot sauce
½ teaspoon ground	Finely chopped onion

1. Use your fingers to pull apart the jackfruit pieces into shreds and place them in a medium pan with a lid. 2. Over medium-high heat, sauté the jackfruit, onion, and garlic with water for 2 minutes. 3. Add cumin, coriander, cinnamon, liquid smoke, and broth, mixing well. 4. Bring the broth to a boil by turning the heat to high, then cover the pan and reduce heat to low. 5. Let it simmer for 15 minutes. 6. Once done, divide the mixture into 8 portions and fill each corn tortilla. Serve with optional toppings or your favorite taco fixings. Enjoy your delicious Jackfruit Carnitas Tacos!

Per Serving:

calories: 265 | fat: 3g | protein: 6g | carbs: 60g | fiber: 6g

Miso Gravy

Prep time: 10 minutes | Cook time: 10 minutes | Serves 12

½ cup whole wheat flour	vinegar
2 garlic cloves, chopped	2 tablespoons maple syrup (optional)
2½ cups water	
½ cup nutritional yeast	2 tablespoons tahini
3 tablespoons red miso	¼ teaspoon black pepper
2 tablespoons apple cider	Salt to taste (optional)

1. Cook flour and garlic in a medium saucepan over medium heat until garlic is soft and flour is toasty (about 3 minutes). 2. Increase heat to medium-high, add water, and whisk constantly until the mixture thickens (about 3 minutes). It should be pourable but may need a spatula's help. 3. Transfer the garlic-flour mixture to a blender, add nutritional yeast, miso, vinegar, maple syrup (if desired), tahini, and pepper. Blend from low to high until well combined. 4. Taste and adjust seasoning as needed, then serve. The gravy can be refrigerated for up to 4 days in an airtight container. Enjoy this flavorful and versatile miso gravy!

Per Serving:

calories: 73 | fat: 2g | protein: 5g | carbs: 10g | fiber: 2g

Chipotle–Pumpkin Seed Salsa

Prep time: 5 minutes | Cook time: 10 minutes | Serves 12

½ cup raw pumpkin seeds	chopped
1 yellow onion, diced	1 (28-ounce / 794-g) can diced tomatoes with juice
3 garlic cloves, minced	
1 or 2 gluten-free chipotles chiles in adobo sauce,	¼ teaspoon salt, plus more to taste (optional)

1. Toast pumpkin seeds in a skillet over low heat until light brown and fragrant (about 3 minutes). Transfer to a bowl and set aside. 2. Increase heat to medium-high, add onions and garlic to the skillet. Cook for about 3 minutes, stirring occasionally. Stir in chipotles and cook for 1 more minute. Add tomatoes with their juice and cook for 5 minutes without stirring. Remove from heat and stir. 3. Place toasted pumpkin seeds in a food processor and pulse until partially ground with some larger pieces. Return them to the bowl. 4. Add the tomato mixture to the food processor, pulse several times, add salt (if desired), and pulse until the salsa is uniform in texture. 5. Transfer the tomato mixture to the bowl with the pumpkin seeds, stir to combine, and season with salt. Serve immediately or refrigerate in an airtight container for up to 3 days. Enjoy this flavorful chipotle-pumpkin seed salsa!

Per Serving:

calories: 44 | fat: 3g | protein: 2g | carbs: 4g | fiber: 2g

Quick Spelt Bread

Prep time: 5 minutes | Cook time: 45 minutes | Makes 1 loaf

420 grams whole-grain spelt flour (about 3¾ cups)	milk
	2 tablespoons pure maple syrup
1 teaspoon baking soda	
1 teaspoon baking powder	1 tablespoon lemon juice
1½ cups unsweetened soy	

1. Preheat your oven to 350ºF (180ºC). 2. Line a 9-by-5-inch loaf pan with parchment paper, ensuring it extends beyond the edges to aid in removing the bread later. 3. In a large bowl, combine spelt flour, baking soda, and baking powder. 4. In a separate medium bowl, mix soy milk, maple syrup, and lemon juice. 5. Add the soy milk mixture to the flour mixture, stirring well until fully combined and the dough starts to form. 6. Transfer the dough to the prepared loaf pan. 7. Bake for approximately 45 minutes until the loaf turns golden brown and a wooden skewer inserted in the center comes out clean. 8. Using the parchment paper sling, remove the bread from the pan, and allow it to cool completely before slicing. Enjoy this quick and delicious spelt bread!

Per Serving:

calories: 204 | fat: 2g | protein: 8g | carbs: 42g | fiber: 6g

Sunflower Parmesan "Cheese"

Prep time: 5 minutes | Cook time: 0 minutes | Makes ½ cup

½ cup sunflower seeds	yeast
2 tablespoons nutritional	½ teaspoon garlic powder

1. In a food processor or blender, combine sunflower seeds, nutritional yeast, and garlic powder. Process on low for 30 to 45 seconds until the sunflower seeds resemble coarse sea salt in size. 2. Transfer the mixture to a refrigerator-safe container and store for up to 2 months. Enjoy this flavorful and dairy-free alternative as a topping for various dishes!

Per Serving: (1 tablespoon)

calories: 56 | fat: 4g | protein: 3g | carbs: 3g | fiber: 1g

Creamy Balsamic Dressing

Prep time: 10 minutes | Cook time: 0 minutes | Makes ¾ cup

¼ cup tahini	(optional)
¼ cup balsamic vinegar	1 garlic clove, pressed
¼ cup fresh basil, minced	Pinch sea salt (optional)
⅛ cup water	Pinch freshly ground black
1 tablespoon maple syrup	pepper (optional)

1. Combine all the ingredients in a blender or food processor and blend until smooth. If you prefer, you can whisk the ingredients together, ensuring the basil is finely minced. Enjoy this delicious dressing on your favorite salads!

Per Serving: (1 tablespoon)

calories: 157 | fat: 10g | protein: 3g | carbs: 12g | fiber: 2g

Oil-Free Sundried Tomato and Oregano Dressing

Prep time: 10 minutes | Cook time: 5 minutes | Makes 3 cups

2 cups filtered water	2 tablespoons pure maple
½ cup sundried tomato	syrup (optional)
halves	¼ teaspoon dried oregano
1 clove garlic, chopped	salt and pepper, to taste
1 small shallot, chopped	(optional)
2 tablespoons Dijon mustard	

1. Bring 2 cups of water to a boil. In a small bowl, combine the sundried tomatoes with the boiling water and let them soften for about 10 minutes. 2. Transfer the softened sundried tomatoes and soaking liquid into a blender. Add garlic, shallots, Dijon mustard, maple syrup, oregano, salt, and optional pepper. Blend the mixture on high until it becomes smooth and creamy. This process may take around 3 minutes, with occasional pauses for scraping down. 3. Store the dressing in the refrigerator for up to 1 week. Enjoy this flavorful, oil-free dressing on your favorite salads or dishes!

Per Serving: (½ cup)

calories: 37 | fat: 0g | protein: 1g | carbs: 8g | fiber: 1g

Beet Dressing

Prep time: 15 minutes | Cook time: 0 minutes | Makes 1 cup

1 small-medium cooked and cooled red beet	vinegar
	2 tablespoons extra-virgin
¼ cup filtered water	olive oil (optional)
3 tablespoons raw cashew butter, coconut butter, or tahini	1 (¼-inch) slice of a large garlic clove
	½ teaspoon fine sea salt, plus
2 tablespoons plus 1 teaspoon raw apple cider	more to taste (optional)

1. In a blender, combine the beet, water, nut or coconut butter or tahini, vinegar, olive oil, garlic, and salt (if using). Blend until smooth, scraping down the sides as needed. Adjust seasoning to taste. 2. Serve immediately or store in a glass jar in the fridge for up to 3 days. Shake well before using, and if it thickens, you can thin it out with a little water if desired. Enjoy this vibrant and flavorful dressing on your salads!

Per Serving: (¼ cup)

calories: 141 | fat: 13g | protein: 3g | carbs: 6g | fiber: 1g

Jalapeño and Tomatillo Salsa

Prep time: 10 minutes | Cook time: 0 minutes | Makes 3 cups

4 tomatillos, peeled and washed	1 garlic clove
	½ bunch fresh cilantro (about
3 jalapeño peppers, stemmed and seeded	1 cup leaves and stems)
	¼ teaspoon salt, plus more
½ medium yellow onion, peeled	as needed (optional)
	1 cup water

1. In a blender, combine the tomatillos, jalapeños, onion, garlic, cilantro, salt (if using), and water. Blend until smooth. Taste and add more salt if desired. Transfer the salsa to an airtight container and store it in the refrigerator for up to 10 days. This zesty and flavorful salsa is perfect for adding a spicy kick to your dishes!

Per Serving:

calories: 7 | fat: 0g | protein: 0g | carbs: 1g | fiber: 0g

Coconut Whipped Cream

Prep time: 5 minutes | Cook time: 0 minutes | Serves 5

1 cup coconut cream	2 tablespoons cocoa powder
1 teaspoon vanilla extract	(optional)

1. In a large bowl, add all the ingredients. Use an electric mixer with beaters or a whisk to mix for about 5 minutes until light and fluffy. 2. Serve the whipped cream chilled as a delicious topping or side. 3. Store the whipped cream in the fridge in an airtight container and consume within 2 days. Alternatively, you can freeze the whipped cream for up to 60 days and thaw at room temperature when needed. Enjoy the creamy and coconutty goodness!

Per Serving:

calories: 40 | fat: 1g | protein: 0g | carbs: 7g | fiber: 0g

Sweet Corn Dressing

Prep time: 10 minutes | Cook time: 0 minutes | Makes 2 cups

2 large ears sweet corn, husked and kernels cut off	white and light green parts only, coarsely chopped
6 tablespoons extra-virgin olive oil (optional)	1 (½-inch) slice of a large garlic clove
¼ cup freshly squeezed lime juice, plus more to taste	¾ teaspoon fine sea salt, plus more to taste (optional)
2 (3-inch) pieces scallion,	

1. Combine corn kernels, olive oil, lime juice, scallion, garlic, and salt (if using) in a blender. Blend until smooth and velvety, scraping down the sides as needed. Adjust seasoning and lime juice to taste and blend again. 2. Serve immediately or store in a glass jar in the fridge for up to 3 days. Shake well before using. Enjoy this flavorful dressing on your salads and dishes!

Per Serving: (¼ cup)

calories: 125 | fat: 10g | protein: 1g | carbs: 8g | fiber: 1g

Italian Spices

Prep time: 5 minutes | Cook time: 0 minutes | Makes ½ cup

¼ cup dried oregano	1 tablespoon garlic powder
3 tablespoons fennel seeds	

1. Combine all the ingredients in a jar with a tight-fitting lid. 2. Shake well to mix. 3. Store the spice blend for up to 6 months, and use it to add delicious Italian flavors to your dishes.

Per Serving: (½ cup)

calories: 132 | fat: 3g | protein: 6g | carbs: 26g | fiber: 14g

Nutty Plant-Based Parmesan

Prep time: 10 minutes | Cook time: 0 minutes | Makes 1½ cups

1 cup raw cashews	½ teaspoon salt (optional)
½ cup nutritional yeast	

1. Pulse the cashews in a blender until they become a fine dust. Transfer the cashew dust to a small bowl and add the nutritional yeast and salt (if using). Mix well with a spoon. Store any leftovers in an airtight container in the refrigerator for up to 10 days or freeze for up to 3 months. This nutty and cheesy topping is a great addition to various dishes!

Per Serving:

calories: 79 | fat: 5g | protein: 3g | carbs: 5g | fiber: 0g

Pineapple Salsa

Prep time: 5 minutes | Cook time: 0 minutes | Serves 8

1 pound (454 g) fresh or thawed frozen pineapple, finely diced, and juices reserved	diced 1 bunch cilantro or mint, leaves only, chopped
1 white or red onion, finely	1 jalapeño, minced (optional) Salt (optional)

1. In a medium bowl, combine the pineapple with its juice, onion, cilantro, and jalapeño, if desired. Season with salt to taste. Serve and enjoy this sweet and tangy salsa with your favorite dishes!

Per Serving:

calories: 40 | fat: 0g | protein: 0g | carbs: 10g | fiber: 1g

Peanut Butter Apple Sauce

Prep time: 10 minutes | Cook time: 15 minutes | Serves 16

4 large apples, peeled and cored	¼ cup raisins 1 tablespoon cinnamon
½ cup peanut butter	½ cup water

1. Cut apples into tiny pieces and cook them in a saucepan with water over low heat until soft. 2. Mash the apples with a fork or potato masher. 3. Stir in peanut butter until well combined. 4. Adjust consistency with more water if needed, then add raisins and cinnamon. 5. Stir thoroughly and serve warm or cold. 6. Store in the fridge (within 3 days) or freezer (up to 60 days) in an airtight container. Enjoy!

Per Serving:

calories: 91 | fat: 4g | protein: 2g | carbs: 12g | fiber: 2g

Quick Mole Sauce

**Prep time: 40 minutes | Cook time: 25 minutes |
Makes 4 cups**

4 dried pasilla chiles
2 dried ancho chiles
Boiling water, for soaking
the peppers
1 yellow onion, cut into
slices
6 garlic cloves, coarsely
chopped
1 tablespoon water, plus
more as needed
2 tablespoons tomato paste
1 jalapeño pepper, seeded
and chopped

2 ounces (57 g) vegan dark
chocolate
2 tablespoons whole wheat
flour
2 tablespoons cocoa powder
2 tablespoons almond butter
2 teaspoons smoked paprika
1 teaspoon ground cumin
1 teaspoon ground cinnamon
½ teaspoon dried oregano
2½ cups no-sodium
vegetable broth

1. Soak pasilla and ancho chiles in boiling water for 20 minutes, then drain. 2. Sauté onion and garlic until dark brown. 3. Blend chiles, jalapeño, chocolate, flour, cocoa powder, almond butter, spices, and vegetable broth until smooth. 4. Simmer the sauce until it bubbles. Serve immediately or store refrigerated/frozen.

Per Serving: (½ cup)
calories: 114 | fat: 7g | protein: 4g | carbs: 13g | fiber: 4g

Creamy Carrot Dressing

**Prep time: 15 minutes | Cook time: 0 minutes |
Makes 1½ cups**

2 medium carrots, chopped
or grated
½ cup filtered water
¼ cup raw cashews
¼ cup extra-virgin olive oil
(optional)
3 tablespoons freshly
squeezed lime juice
1 (3-inch) piece scallion,

white and light green parts
only, coarsely chopped
1 (½-inch) slice of a large
garlic clove
½ teaspoon fine sea salt, plus
more to taste (optional)
1 teaspoon tamari, plus more
to taste

1. In an upright blender, combine the carrots, water, cashews, olive oil, lime juice, scallion, garlic, salt (if using), and tamari. Blend until the mixture is completely smooth and creamy, which may take about 1 minute. Scrape down the sides of the blender with a rubber spatula and blend again. Adjust the seasoning to taste and blend once more. 2. Serve the dressing immediately, or store it in a glass jar in the fridge for up to 3 days. Before using, shake the jar well as the dressing may thicken once chilled. If needed, you can thin it out with a little water. Enjoy this delicious and nutritious dressing on salads, vegetables, or as a dip!

Per Serving: (¼ cup)
calories: 124 | fat: 11g | protein: 2g | carbs: 5g | fiber: 1g

Mocha-Walnut Cashew Butter

**Prep time: 10 minutes | Cook time: 20 minutes |
Makes 2 cups**

2 cups raw cashews
1 cup raw walnuts
3 tablespoons cacao powder
2 tablespoons pure maple
syrup (optional)

1 teaspoon vanilla extract
1 teaspoon instant coffee
grounds or espresso powder
2 tablespoons nut-based oil
(optional)

1. Preheat the oven to 350ºF (180ºC). 2. Spread the cashews and walnuts on a baking sheet and bake for 10 minutes. Shake the sheet, then bake for 5 to 10 minutes more until golden brown. Let cool for 15 minutes. 3. Transfer the toasted nuts to a food processor or high-speed blender. Add the cacao powder, maple syrup (if using), vanilla, and instant coffee. Process until crumbly, scrape down the sides, and continue to process until smooth. The amount of time it takes for your nut butter to go from a thick ball to creamy smooth depends on your equipment. A high-speed blender might take only 2 minutes, whereas a food processor can take up to 10 minutes. 4. Transfer to a sealable container like a widemouthed mason jar.

Per Serving: (1 tablespoon)
calories: 72 | fat: 6g | protein: 2g | carbs: 4g | fiber: 1g

Vegan Basil Pesto

Prep time: 5 minutes | Cook time: 0 minutes | Serves 6

2 bunches basil, leaves only
1 cup spinach
¼ cup roasted almonds
¼ cup toasted pine nuts
4 raw Brazil nuts, chopped

2 garlic cloves
¼ cup water
¼ to ½ teaspoon salt
(optional)

1. In a food processor, pulse the basil, spinach, almonds, pine nuts, Brazil nuts, and garlic until finely chopped and combined. While the processor is running, stream in water until you achieve your desired consistency. Add ¼ teaspoon salt, then adjust to taste if desired. 2. Store the pesto in an airtight container in the refrigerator for up to 5 days. For longer storage, freeze in single portions by scooping into ice cube trays, freezing, and then transferring to an airtight container. Enjoy this flavorful and versatile vegan pesto in various dishes!

Per Serving:
calories: 81 | fat: 8g | protein: 2g | carbs: 2g | fiber: 1g

Refrigerator Pickles

Prep time: 20 minutes | Cook time: 10 minutes | Makes 2 pints

1 pound (454 g) small cucumbers, preferably pickling cucumbers, washed and dried	1 cup apple cider vinegar
	1 cup water
	¼ cup beet sugar (optional)
	1 tablespoon kosher salt (optional)
1 small yellow onion, chopped or cut into rings	1 tablespoon pickling spice

1. Using a sharp knife or mandoline, slice the unpeeled cucumbers into ¼-inch-thick rounds. 2. In a large bowl, mix the cucumbers and onions. Divide the mixture between two widemouthed 1-pint canning jars with lids, packing them in gently. Leave ½ inch of headspace at the top of the jars. 3. In a small pot over high heat, combine the vinegar, water, beet sugar, salt (if using), and pickling spice. Bring to a boil, stirring until the sugar and salt dissolve. Pour the brine over the vegetables, leaving ½ inch of headspace. If needed, add more brine to fill the jars to the ½-inch line, then secure the lids tightly. Let the jars cool to room temperature. 4. Refrigerate for at least 24 hours before serving. These pickles will develop more flavor over time and maintain a crisp texture. 5. Due to the high acid content in the brine, you can keep these pickles refrigerated for 1 month or longer, but they are not shelf-stable since they were not canned. Enjoy these delicious homemade pickles as a crunchy and tangy addition to your meals!

Per Serving: (4 pickles)

calories: 218 | fat: 1g | protein: 4g | carbs: 50g | fiber: 7g

Cheesy Vegetable Sauce

Prep time: 10 minutes | Cook time: 25 minutes | Makes 4 cups

1 cup raw cashews	(or almond or cashew if gluten-free)
1 russet potato, peeled and cubed	1 tablespoon arrowroot powder, cornstarch, or tapioca starch
2 carrots, cubed	
½ cup nutritional yeast	
2 tablespoons yellow (mellow) miso paste	1 onion, chopped
	3 garlic cloves, minced
1 teaspoon ground mustard	1 tablespoon water, plus more as needed
2 cups unsweetened oat milk	

1. In an 8-quart pot, combine the cashews, potato, and carrots. Add enough water to cover by 2 inches. Bring to a boil over high heat, then reduce the heat to simmer. Cook for 15 minutes. 2. In a blender, combine the nutritional yeast, miso paste, ground mustard, milk, and arrowroot powder. 3. Drain the cashews, potato, and carrot. Add to the blender but don't blend yet. 4. Rinse the pot, place it over high heat, and add the onion and garlic. Cook for 3 to 4 minutes, adding water 1 tablespoon at a time to prevent burning. Transfer to the blender. Purée everything until smooth. Scrape the

sides and continue blending as needed. Pour the cheese sauce into the pot and place it over medium heat. Cook, stirring, until the sauce comes to a simmer. 5. Use immediately, or refrigerate in a sealable container for up to 1 week.

Per Serving: (½ cup)

calories: 191 | fat: 10g | protein: 9g | carbs: 20g | fiber: 4g

Green Goddess Dressing

Prep time: 10 minutes | Cook time: 0 minutes | Makes 1 cup

½ cup tahini	½ cup fresh parsley, minced
2 tablespoons apple cider vinegar	½ cup scallions or chives, minced
Juice of 1 lemon	¼ teaspoon sea salt (optional)
¼ cup tamari or soy sauce	
2 garlic cloves, minced or pressed	Pinch freshly ground black pepper (optional)
½ cup water	1 tablespoon maple syrup (optional)
½ cup fresh basil, minced	

1. Put all the ingredients into a blender or food processor and blend until smooth for about 30 to 45 seconds. If the consistency is too thick, add more water until you achieve a creamy dressing. Enjoy!

Per Serving: (1 tablespoon)

calories: 211 | fat: 16g | protein: 7g | carbs: 12g | fiber: 1g

Flavorful Vegetable Broth

Prep time: 5 minutes | Cook time: 50 minutes | Makes 4 quarts

4½ quarts water	½ teaspoon black peppercorns
2 medium onions, quartered	
3 cups chopped celery	4 bay leaves
3 cups chopped carrots	1 cup chopped fennel bulb (optional)
4 large garlic cloves, minced	
1 tablespoon chopped fresh rosemary	1 ounce (28 g) dried wild mushrooms (optional)
2 teaspoons dried thyme	

1. Combine water, onions, celery, carrots, garlic, herbs, peppercorns, bay leaves, and optional fennel and mushrooms in a large pot. Bring to a boil, then cover and simmer on low for 45 minutes. 2. Strain the broth through a coffee filter or cheesecloth-lined strainer into a large bowl. 3. Transfer the strained broth into glass jars, seal, and refrigerate for up to 7 days or freeze for up to 6 months. Enjoy this delicious and versatile broth in your favorite recipes!

Per Serving:

calories: 15 | fat: 0g | protein: 1g | carbs: 3g | fiber: 1g

Cauliflower Bake Topping

Prep time: 10 minutes | Cook time: 15 minutes | Serves 6

1 large head cauliflower, cut into 1½-inch florets ½ cup raw pine nuts, cashews, or macadamia nuts ½ cup filtered water if using a food processor	2 tablespoons extra-virgin olive oil (optional) 3 tablespoons nutritional yeast, plus more to taste ½ teaspoon fine sea salt, plus more to taste (optional)

1. Set up a steamer pot with about 2 inches of filtered water in the bottom (the water shouldn't touch the bottom of the basket) and bring to a boil over high heat. Arrange the cauliflower florets in the steamer basket, cover, and steam for 10 to 12 minutes, until the cauliflower is cooked through but not falling apart. Remove from the heat and set aside. 2. High-Powered-Blender Method: Put the nuts, olive oil, yeast, and salt, if using, in a high-powered blender and add the steamed cauliflower. Starting on low speed and using the tamper stick to help press the cauliflower down, blend, gradually increasing the speed to high, until completely smooth and thick; use the tamper stick to keep the mixture moving and to scrape down the sides as you go. This will take a couple of minutes. Season with more nutritional yeast and salt to taste and blend to combine. 3. Food-Processor Method: Put the steamed cauliflower in a food processor. Combine the nuts, water, olive oil, yeast, and salt in a regular upright blender and blend until completely smooth. Pour into the food processor with the cauliflower and process until completely smooth, scraping down the sides as necessary. Season with more yeast and salt to taste. 4. The topping is ready to be baked on a filling of your choice, or it can be stored in an airtight container in the fridge for up to 3 days or frozen for up to 3 months.

Per Serving:

calories: 167 | fat: 13g | protein: 6g | carbs: 10g | fiber: 4g

Perfect Marinara Sauce

Prep time: 10 minutes | Cook time: 20 minutes | Makes 7 cups

2 (28-ounce / 794-g) cans crushed tomatoes in purée 4 garlic cloves, minced 2 tablespoons Italian seasoning 2 teaspoons pure maple	syrup 2 teaspoons onion powder 2 teaspoons paprika ¼ teaspoon freshly ground black pepper

1. In a medium saucepan, stir together the tomatoes, garlic, Italian seasoning, maple syrup, onion powder, paprika, and pepper. Bring to a simmer. 2. Reduce the heat to low. Cover, and simmer for 15 to 20 minutes, or until the sauce is fragrant and the flavors have melded together. Remove from the heat.

Per Serving:

calories: 39 | fat: 0g | protein: 2g | carbs: 8g | fiber: 2g

Korean Tahini BBQ Sauce

Prep time: 10 minutes | Cook time: 0 minutes | Makes ¾ cup

½ cup water ¼ cup red miso 1 piece ginger, peeled and minced	3 cloves garlic, minced 2 tablespoons chili paste or chili sauce 2 tablespoons rice vinegar 2 tablespoons tahini

1. Purée all the ingredients in a mini blender until smooth. Serve as is or thin with an additional ½ cup water and use as a marinade for tofu, tempeh, or portobello mushroom caps.

Per Serving: (¼ cup)

calories: 124 | fat: 7g | protein: 5g | carbs: 12g | fiber: 3g

Whipped Coconut Cream

Prep time: 5 minutes | Cook time: 0 minutes | Makes 1 cup

1 can (13½ ounces / 383 g) full-fat coconut milk, chilled overnight
1 tablespoon pure maple syrup (optional)
½ teaspoon pure vanilla extract

1. Remove the chilled can of coconut milk from the refrigerator. When you open it, there should be a thick layer of pure coconut cream on top. Scoop this coconut cream into a medium bowl, being careful to avoid the water at the bottom of the can. Reserve the water for smoothies or discard. 2. To the coconut cream, add the maple syrup and vanilla and whisk vigorously by hand until you have a smooth and light cream. You could also whip this in a blender, food processor, or with a hand mixer.

Per Serving: (¼ cup)

calories: 235 | fat: 22g | protein: 2g | carbs: 9g | fiber: 2g

Raw Date Paste

Prep time: 10 minutes | Cook time: 0 minutes | Makes 2½ cups

1 cup Medjool dates, pitted and chopped
1½ cups water

1. In a blender, combine the dates and water, and blend until you have a smooth paste. 2. Transfer the date paste to an airtight container and store it in the refrigerator. It will stay fresh for up to 7 days. This delicious and natural sweetener can be used in various recipes or enjoyed on its own as a healthy alternative to refined sugar.

Per Serving:

calories: 21 | fat: 0g | protein: 0g | carbs: 5g | fiber: 1g

Roasted Beet Dip

Prep time: 5 minutes | Cook time: 30 to 40 minutes | Makes 2 cups

2 medium or 3 small red beets	2 tablespoons balsamic vinegar
½ cup sunflower seeds, soaked in water for 8 hours	1 teaspoon fennel seeds
1 tablespoon hemp oil (optional)	½ teaspoon sea salt (optional)
Juice of 1 lemon	½ teaspoon freshly ground black pepper

1. Preheat your oven to 400ºF (205ºC). Wrap the beets in unbleached parchment paper and place them on a baking sheet. Roast for 30 to 40 minutes until the beets are tender when pierced with a fork. 2. Once the beets are cool enough to handle, peel away the skins using your hands. Chop the beets and place them in a blender or food processor. Add the remaining ingredients and blend until smooth. 3. Transfer the dip to an airtight container and store it in the refrigerator for up to 5 days. Enjoy this delicious and nutritious Roasted Beet Dip as a flavorful spread for sandwiches, a dip for veggies or crackers, or a tasty addition to your weekday lunches and snacks.

Per Serving:
calories: 81 | fat: 6g | protein: 2g | carbs: 4g | fiber: 1g

Vegetable Broth

Prep time: 20 minutes | Cook time: 40 minutes | Serves 10

10 cups water	½ cup fresh parsley
2 onions, chopped	½ cup olive oil (optional)
3 medium cloves garlic, minced	1 tablespoon miso paste
4 carrots, chopped	2 tablespoons nutritional yeast (optional)
3 leafless celery ribs, chopped	1 thyme
1 sweet potato, cubed	1 tablespoon rosemary
1 red bell pepper, sliced	Salt and black pepper to taste (optional)
1 cup fresh or frozen kale	

1. Preheat your oven to 400ºF (205ºC). 2. Toss onions, garlic, carrots, celery, sweet potato, bell pepper, kale, and parsley with ½ cup of olive oil in an oven-proof roasting pan or baking tray. Roast the vegetables in the oven for approximately 20 minutes until they are browned and caramelized. 3. In a large pot, bring about 10 cups of water to a boil. Add all the roasted vegetables to the pot with the boiling water. Reduce the heat to low, maintaining a gentle simmer. Stir occasionally, and then add miso paste, nutritional yeast, thyme, and rosemary. Season with salt, pepper, and any other desired spices to taste. Let it simmer until about half of the water has evaporated. Remove the pot from the stove and allow it to cool slightly. 4. Pour the mixture through a sieve, collecting the flavorful broth in a second pot. Serve immediately as a delicious and nutritious base for soups, stews, or other dishes. Enjoy the rich flavors of this homemade vegetable broth!

Per Serving:
calories: 143 | fat: 11g | protein: 2g | carbs: 10g | fiber: 2g

Almond-Lemon Ricotta

Prep time: 5 minutes | Cook time: 0 minutes | Makes 1 cup

2 cups blanched slivered almonds (not sliced)	1 tablespoon lemon zest
¾ cup cold water	1 tablespoon pure maple syrup (optional)
2 tablespoons freshly squeezed lemon juice	2 teaspoons nutritional yeast
	½ teaspoon almond extract

1. In a food processor or high-speed blender, combine the almonds, water, lemon juice, lemon zest, maple syrup (if using), nutritional yeast, and almond extract. Pulse to combine, scrape down the sides, and purée until mostly smooth. 2. Refrigerate in an airtight container for up to 2 weeks, or freeze for up to 6 months.

Per Serving: (2 tablespoons)
calories: 166 | fat: 14g | protein: 6g | carbs: 8g | fiber: 4g

Toasted Seed and Nori Salad Topper

Prep time: 10 minutes | Cook time: 20 minutes | Makes 2 cups

½ cup raw pumpkin seeds	1 teaspoon tamari
½ cup raw unhulled sesame seeds	½ teaspoon fine sea salt (optional)
½ cup raw sunflower seeds	¼ teaspoon cayenne pepper
1 teaspoon raw apple cider vinegar	⅛ teaspoon garlic powder
	½ cup crushed nori

1. Preheat the oven to 300ºF (150ºC). Line a rimmed baking sheet with parchment paper and set aside. 2. Put the pumpkin, sesame, and sunflower seeds in a medium strainer and rinse under cold running water. Set aside to drain well. 3. Transfer the drained seeds to a medium bowl and add the vinegar, tamari, salt, cayenne, and garlic powder, if using. Mix well, then spread the seeds out on the lined baking sheet in a single layer. Toast for 10 minutes, stir, and toast for another 6 to 8 minutes, until the seeds are fragrant and golden. Remove from the oven and set aside to cool. 4. Transfer the seeds to a dry bowl, add the nori flakes, and mix well. Store in an airtight jar for up to 6 weeks.

Per Serving: (⅛ cup)
calories: 156 | fat: 14g | protein: 6g | carbs: 5g | fiber: 2g

Everyday Pesto

Prep time: 5 minutes | Cook time: 5 minutes | Makes 1 cup

4 cups packed fresh basil leaves	1 garlic clove
¼ cup raw cashews	¼ teaspoon freshly ground black pepper
2 tablespoons nutritional yeast	3 tablespoons boiling water, plus more as needed

1. In a food processor, blend the basil, cashews, nutritional yeast, garlic, pepper, and boiling water until smooth. Add more water to thin until you have a smooth, slightly thick mixture. 2. Refrigerate in a sealed jar for up to 1 month.

Per Serving: (2 tablespoons)

calories: 35 | fat: 2g | protein: 3g | carbs: 2g | fiber: 1g

Nut Milk

Prep time: 5 minutes | Cook time: 0 minutes | Makes 5 cups

1 cup raw cashews or almonds, soaked overnight and drained	1 teaspoon vanilla extract (optional)
3 dates, pitted (optional)	4 cups water

1. In a blender combine the soaked nuts, dates (if using), vanilla (if using), and water and blend on high for 3 to 4 minutes, until the nuts are all pulverized and the liquid looks creamy. 2. Pour the blended mix through a nut milk bag, cheesecloth, or a fine-mesh sieve and pour it into an airtight storage container. Chill and use within 4 days.

Per Serving:

calories: 25 | fat: 2g | protein: 0g | carbs: 1g | fiber: 0g

Roasted Jalapeño and Lime Guacamole

Prep time: 5 minutes | Cook time: 10 minutes | Serves 4

1 to 3 jalapeños	1 tablespoon freshly squeezed lime juice
1 avocado, peeled and pitted	

1. Preheat the oven to 400°F (205°C). Line a baking sheet with parchment paper. 2. Place the jalapeños on the baking sheet and roast for 8 minutes. (The jalapeño can also be roasted on a grill for 5 minutes, if you already have it fired up.) 3. Slice the jalapeños down the center, and remove the seeds. Then cut the top stem off, and dice into ⅛-inch pieces. Wash your hands immediately after handling the jalapeños. 4. In a medium bowl, use a fork to mash together the avocado, jalapeño pieces, and lime juice. Continue mashing and mixing until the guacamole reaches your preferred consistency, and serve.

Per Serving:

calories: 77 | fat: 7g | protein: 1g | carbs: 5g | fiber: 3g

Artichoke Dressing

Prep time: 10 minutes | Cook time: 0 minutes | Makes 1 cup

1 cup drained jarred or canned artichoke hearts	1 tablespoon freshly squeezed lemon juice, plus more to taste
1 (3-inch) piece scallion, white and light green parts only, coarsely chopped	6 tablespoons filtered water
¼ cup extra-virgin olive oil (optional)	½ teaspoon fine sea salt, plus more to taste (optional)

1. Combine the artichokes, scallion, olive oil, lemon juice, water, and salt, if using, in an upright blender and blend until completely smooth. Scrape down the sides with a rubber spatula and blend again. Adjust the seasoning and lemon juice to taste and blend again. 2. Serve immediately, or store in a glass jar in the fridge for up to 3 days. Shake well before using.

Per Serving: (¼ cup)

calories: 144 | fat: 14g | protein: 1g | carbs: 6g | fiber: 4g

Jerk Spices

Prep time: 5 minutes | Cook time: 0 minutes | Makes ⅓ cup

1 tablespoon garlic powder	½ teaspoon crushed red pepper
2 teaspoons dried thyme	¼ teaspoon cumin seeds
2 teaspoons onion powder	¼ teaspoon freshly grated nutmeg
1 teaspoon black pepper	¼ teaspoon ground cinnamon
1 teaspoon dried parsley	
1 teaspoon sweet paprika	
1 teaspoon whole allspice	
½ teaspoon cayenne pepper	

1. Pulse all the ingredients in a clean coffee grinder until thoroughly combined. Store in an airtight container for up to 6 months.

Per Serving: (⅓ cup)

calories: 83 | fat: 1g | protein: 3g | carbs: 18g | fiber: 5g

Super-Simple Guacamole

Prep time: 10 minutes | Cook time: 0 minutes | Makes 1½ cups

2 avocados, peeled and pitted
Juice of ½ lime
Pinch of salt (optional)
2 tablespoons chopped fresh

cilantro
1 tomato, chopped
1 scallion, white and green parts, chopped

1. In a medium bowl, combine the avocados, lime juice, and salt (if using) and mash together until it reaches your desired consistency. Add the cilantro, tomato, and scallion and mix well. Serve immediately.

Per Serving:

calories: 113 | fat: 10g | protein: 2g | carbs: 7g | fiber: 5g

Chimichurri

Prep time: 5 minutes | Cook time: 0 minutes | Serves 6

1 cup flat-leaf parsley leaves
Grated zest and juice of 2 lemons

4 garlic cloves
1 teaspoon dried oregano
¼ cup water

1. Pulse the parsley, lemon zest and juice, garlic, and oregano in a food processor until combined. With the food processor running, stream in the water, stopping when it reaches the desired consistency. 2. The chimichurri can be refrigerated in an airtight container for up to 5 days. It can also be frozen in single portions for up to 6 months: Scoop into ice cube trays, freeze, then transfer to an airtight container.

Per Serving:

calories: 11 | fat: 0g | protein: 1g | carbs: 3g | fiber: 1g

Italian Seasoning

Prep time: 5 minutes | Cook time: 0 minutes | Makes 9 tablespoons

8 teaspoons dried marjoram
8 teaspoons dried basil
4 teaspoons dried thyme
2 teaspoons dried rosemary

2 teaspoons dried sage
2 teaspoons dried oregano
1 teaspoon garlic powder

1. In an airtight container with a lid (or repurposed spice jar), combine the marjoram, basil, thyme, rosemary, sage, oregano, and garlic powder. Shake or mix well.

Per Serving:

calories: 7 | fat: 0g | protein: 0g | carbs: 2g | fiber: 1g

Smoked Cashew Cheese Spread

Prep time: 5 minutes | Cook time: 0 minutes | Makes 1 cup

1 cup raw cashews
3 cups water
2 garlic cloves
1 tablespoon freshly squeezed lemon juice

¼ teaspoon freshly ground black pepper
½ tablespoon smoked paprika

1. Place the cashews in a small bowl, cover with the water, and soak at room temperature for 2 hours or up to 8 hours. 2. Strain the water from the cashews into another bowl and reserve the liquid for later. 3. Place the soaked cashews in a food processor and add the garlic, lemon juice, pepper, and smoked paprika. Add 2 tablespoons of the strained cashew water and blend to a smooth consistency. Add more water from the soaked nuts if needed.

Per Serving:

calories: 105 | fat: 8g | protein: 3g | carbs: 6g | fiber: 1g

Appendix 1: Measurement Conversion Chart

MEASUREMENT CONVERSION CHART

VOLUME EQUIVALENTS(DRY)

US STANDARD	METRIC (APPROXIMATE)
1/8 teaspoon	0.5 mL
1/4 teaspoon	1 mL
1/2 teaspoon	2 mL
3/4 teaspoon	4 mL
1 teaspoon	5 mL
1 tablespoon	15 mL
1/4 cup	59 mL
1/2 cup	118 mL
3/4 cup	177 mL
1 cup	235 mL
2 cups	475 mL
3 cups	700 mL
4 cups	1 L

VOLUME EQUIVALENTS(LIQUID)

US STANDARD	US STANDARD (OUNCES)	METRIC (APPROXIMATE)
2 tablespoons	1 fl.oz.	30 mL
1/4 cup	2 fl.oz.	60 mL
1/2 cup	4 fl.oz.	120 mL
1 cup	8 fl.oz.	240 mL
1 1/2 cup	12 fl.oz.	355 mL
2 cups or 1 pint	16 fl.oz.	475 mL
4 cups or 1 quart	32 fl.oz.	1 L
1 gallon	128 fl.oz.	4 L

TEMPERATURES EQUIVALENTS

FAHRENHEIT(F)	CELSIUS(C) (APPROXIMATE)
225 °F	107 °C
250 °F	120 °C
275 °F	135 °C
300 °F	150 °C
325 °F	160 °C
350 °F	180 °C
375 °F	190 °C
400 °F	205 °C
425 °F	220 °C
450 °F	235 °C
475 °F	245 °C
500 °F	260 °C

WEIGHT EQUIVALENTS

US STANDARD	METRIC (APPROXIMATE)
1 ounce	28 g
2 ounces	57 g
5 ounces	142 g
10 ounces	284 g
15 ounces	425 g
16 ounces (1 pound)	455 g
1.5 pounds	680 g
2 pounds	907 g

Appendix 2: The Dirty Dozen and Clean Fifteen

The Dirty Dozen and Clean Fifteen

The Environmental Working Group (EWG) is a nonprofit, nonpartisan organization dedicated to protecting human health and the environment Its mission is to empower people to live healthier lives in a healthier environment. This organization publishes an annual list of the twelve kinds of produce, in sequence, that have the highest amount of pesticide residue-the Dirty Dozen-as well as a list of the fifteen kinds ofproduce that have the least amount of pesticide residue-the Clean Fifteen.

THE DIRTY DOZEN	THE CLEAN FIFTEEN
• The 2016 Dirty Dozen includes the following produce. These are considered among the year's most important produce to buy organic:	• The least critical to buy organically are the Clean Fifteen list. The following are on the 2016 list:

THE DIRTY DOZEN

Strawberries	Spinach
Apples	Tomatoes
Nectarines	Bell peppers
Peaches	Cherry tomatoes
Celery	Cucumbers
Grapes	Kale/collard greens
Cherries	Hot peppers

• *The Dirty Dozen list contains two additional itemskale/collard greens and hot peppers-because they tend to contain trace levels of highly hazardous pesticides.*

THE CLEAN FIFTEEN

Avocados	Papayas
Corn	Kiw
Pineapples	Eggplant
Cabbage	Honeydew
Sweet peas	Grapefruit
Onions	Cantaloupe
Asparagus	Cauliflower
Mangos	

• *Some of the sweet corn sold in the United States are made from genetically engineered (GE) seedstock. Buy organic varieties of these crops to avoid GE produce.*

Made in the USA
Las Vegas, NV
14 October 2023

79080437R00063